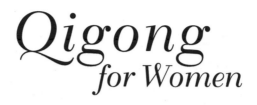

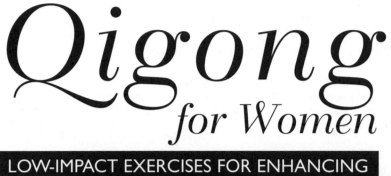

Qigong
for Women

**LOW-IMPACT EXERCISES FOR ENHANCING
ENERGY AND TONING THE BODY**

Dominique Ferraro

translated by Tami Calliope

Healing Arts Press
Rochester, Vermont

Healing Arts Press
One Park Street
Rochester, Vermont 05767
www.InnerTraditions.com

Healing Arts Press is a division of Inner Traditions International

Translation copyright © 2000 by Inner Traditions International
First English language edition published in 2000 by Inner Traditions International
First published in Italian under the title *Qi Gong per la donna* in 1997 by Xenia Edizioni,
Via Carducci 31, Milano, Italy

*Note to the reader: This book is intended as an informational guide. The remedies, approaches, and techniques
described herein are meant to supplement, and not to be a substitute for, professional medical care or treatment.
They should not be used to treat a serious ailment without prior consultation with a qualified health care professional.*

Library of Congress Cataloging-in-Publication Data

Ferraro, Dominique.
   [Qi Gong per la donna. English]
   Qigong for women : low-impact exercises for enhancing energy and toning the body /
Dominique Ferraro.
      p. cm.
   Includes index.
   ISBN 978-0-89281-838-9 (alk. paper)
    1. Ch'i kung.   2. Exercise.   3. Women—Health and hygiene.   I. Title.
   RA781.8 .F477 1999
   613.7'1'082—dc21   99-048331

Printed and bound in India

10 9 8 7 6 5 4 3 2

Text design and layout by Rachel Goldenberg

This book was typeset in Berkeley Book with Post Antiqua as the display typeface.

Acknowledgments

I thank my teachers, both women and men, for their valuable instruction, which has made this book possible: Dr. Ma Xu Zhou, Dr. Zhao Hui Lin, Dr. Grace Yu, Dr. Zang Fu Sheng, Dr. Pang Yin Wu and teacher Mas Rodgers, and Dr. Yves Réquéna.

Dedication

I dedicate this book to all my women students, whose enthusiasm so helped me with this research: Anna, Carla, Caterina, Bruna, Beatrice, Carmela, Cettina, Christiane, Elena, Eva, Francesca, Giancarla, Giuliana, Graziella, Lucia, Marina, Mariolina, Maria Luisa, Micaella, Patrizia, Paola, Piera, Nicole, Raffaella, Silvana, Tiziana, Wanda, and Yvonne.

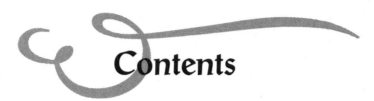

Contents

List of Tables and Figures

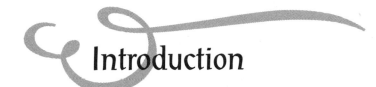

Introduction

What Is Qigong?

Qi (also spelled *chi*) in Chinese means "vital energy," *gong* (or *kung*), "practice" or "exercise." *Qigong* is therefore the technique that allows one to nourish and circulate vital energy to attain physical and psychic well-being and to increase resistance to stress and disease.

Developed and enriched for more than two thousand years—by monks and by doctors, by Taoists and by Buddhists—qigong is a gentle therapeutic exercise, both curative and preventive, based on the ancient system of acupuncture meridians. This "gymnastics of the meridians" comprises both static and dynamic physical exercises, techniques for breath control and mental concentration, self-administered massage and acupressure on acupuncture points, and therapeutic sounds causing vibrations that stimulate different internal organs. The purpose of these exercises is to prevent or dissolve blockages of energy, stimulate the circulation, and correct imbalances. The result is increased psychic and physical well-being and a marked strengthening of immune defenses. With focused practice, any disturbance can be prevented or cured.

Qigong for Today's Women

The woman of today is frequently exposed to frenetic rhythms and heavy psychological pressures. When young she is on the run from morning to night; between housework, career, and family, she has little time to devote to herself, accumulating tensions and stress that begin to manifest themselves in chronic disturbances. As she ages she finds herself a victim to aches and pains that she has been unable either to prevent or to cure, suffering from low morale and low self-esteem and bereft of the enthusiasm necessary to create new interests. She is ashamed of her body, and looking in the mirror becomes discouraging. Depression, often accompanied by other very negative emotions long accumulated and suppressed, assails her, giving rise to any number of serious illnesses.

Yet a solution exists, for both young and elderly women. All it takes is a quarter of an hour a day of practice to attain health, serenity, and a trim figure.

By practicing qigong young women will discover techniques with which to free themselves from tensions and chronic disturbances, keep their bodies fit and healthy, and sustain tranquillity. Middle-aged and elderly women, on the other hand, will recover elasticity, both in their joints and in a newly positive attitude regarding their own lives and futures, learning how to face aging with the strength that comes from a healthy body and a calm and serene mind.

The Principles of Traditional Chinese Medicine

According to Chinese medicine, our bodies contain a dense network of channels that distribute the qi energy among our various organs, allowing communication between them. This network—a fourth separate system in addition to the circulatory, nervous, and lymphatic systems—is invisible but real; it has been tracked by modern instruments that measure variations of electrical resistance on the skin. In today's language it could be said that this network is the information circuit that "keeps it all together," allowing the body's different organs to communicate with one another.

Chinese theory states that any loss of balance or blockage of energy in a given organ has repercussions on all the others, resulting in a general imbalance. The basic principle of Chinese medicine is just this: The corporal system is a unified system, and what is more, the mind and body form a single system; just like colds or viruses, "bad" emotions are pathogens. The therapy for each specific problem, then, aims at reestablishing a comprehensive balance and well-being; one cannot cure the body "piece by piece," as many Western doctors believe. In fact, after Western practitioners have resolved a problem, they often discover that they have provoked another.

Along the outermost reach of this network of channels—the twelve principal meridians and eight extraordinary vessels—are found the acupuncture points, "switches" on which one may act to accelerate or slow energetic circulation in the meridian or to stimulate or soothe an organ. Such points, usually sensitive to pressure and at times quite painful, were discovered empirically in very ancient times, when Chinese shamans undertook to manipulate them with massage, then with splinters of stone or the heat of live embers. Today we use digital acupressure, needles, electrical stimulation, or twigs of *moxa*, a variety of artemisia also called Chinese mugwort, rolled tightly and set alight.

Some meridians are linked precisely to one particular organ, whereas others regulate energetic circulation throughout the body. For an idea of their layout, consult the figures at the end of this book.

Yin and Yang. To understand the Chinese view of the energetic system, one might usefully compare it to electricity: For the current to flow there must be two poles, one negative and the other positive. In this same way each of our organs contains bipolar energies: *yin,* the negative pole, and *yang,* the positive pole. To function well, each organ must receive a sufficient supply of energy in which yin and yang are fully balanced.

The purpose of qigong, like that of acupuncture or Chinese massage, is to bring harmony to the energies in the organs in such a way as to protect the body from attack by external factors (viruses, cold, heat, humidity) as well as internal factors (negative emotions). Every long-standing disequilibrium upsets the energetic circulation, which follows a precise order of influence from organ to organ. These interactions include the spirit, since spirit brings every emotion into rapport with the organ in which it is reflected or by which it is influenced (see Table 1). This general coordination is illustrated by the theory, or rather, the "model," of the Five Elements (Figure 1).

The Theory of the Five Elements. According to ancient Chinese philosophy, the model of the Five Elements reflects the universal law regulating

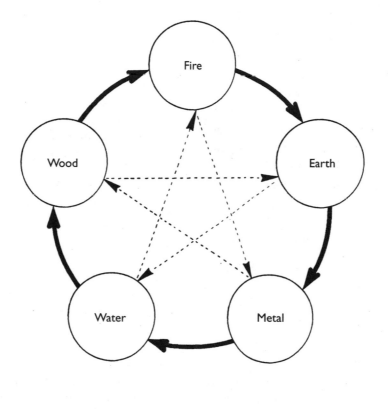

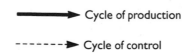 Cycle of production

- - - - -▶ Cycle of control

Figure 1: The cycle of the five elements

the cosmos, nature, and human beings and their health. The Five Elements are symbols of the five fundamental phases of yin/yang transformation.

One is in good health only when one is able to harmonize yin and yang both inside and outside the body, that is, when one is in perfect tune with the environment and nature. In classic symbology human beings are represented as intermediate between sky and earth: We are nourished by air, food, and water and absorb the yang energy of the sky and the yin energy of the earth. Life is based on this continual process of the transformation of energies from different sources.

Each of the principal five yin organs—liver, heart, spleen, lungs, and kidneys—and their corresponding yang organs—gall bladder, small intestine, stomach, large intestine, and urinary bladder—is linked to a symbolic element:

Wood	Fire	Earth	Metal	Water
Liver	Heart	Spleen	Lungs	Kidneys

The order follows a cycle of production: water, by nourishing plants, produces wood, which feeds fire, which produces earth, which produces metal, which in its turn produces water, and so forth. In this "mother-child" law of yin/yang transformation, every movement generates the movement to follow. The corresponding organs are subject to the same principle: the kidneys ("mother") pass along the energy to the liver ("child"), which becomes in turn the "mother" of the heart, to which it will then pass along energy, and so forth.

A cycle of control also exists, the function of which is to compensate for any excesses and imbalances between the various movements. According to this law of inhibition, water quenches fire, which melts metal, which cuts wood, which restrains earth, which holds in water (see Figure 1).

Organization of the Meridians. There are six yang meridians, and the first five on the list are associated with the hollow organs. In addition, one of the two primary extraordinary vessels is yang. The seven major yang channels are:

- The gall bladder meridian (GB)
- The small intestine meridian (SI)
- The stomach meridian (St)
- The large intestine meridian (LI)
- The bladder meridian (B)
- The triple heater meridian (TH)
- The Du Mai, or governing vessel (DM)

There are six yin meridians, and the first five on the list are associated with the principal, or "solid," organs. In addition, the other primary extraordinary vessel is yin. The seven major yin channels are:

- The liver meridian (Lv)
- The heart meridian (H)
- The lung meridian (Lu)
- The spleen meridian (Sp)
- The kidney meridian (K)
- The pericardium meridian (P)
- The Ren Mai, or conception vessel (RM)

The two extraordinary vessels, Ren Mai and Du Mai, which follow the median line of the body on the front and back, are not connected to any particular organ but instead communicate with the totality of the other meridians. Each of the six yang meridians communicates with an associated yin meridian by way of a linking channel called *luo*. The principal meridians and vessels are therefore paired in couples in the following manner:

- Large intestine / lung
- Stomach / spleen
- Small intestine / heart
- Bladder / kidney
- Triple heater / pericardium
- Gall bladder / liver
- Du Mai / Ren Mai

Table I: Correspondences of the Five Elements					
Element	Wood	Fire	Earth	Metal	Water
Color	green	red	yellow	white	black
Direction	east	south	center	west	north
Climate	wind	heat	humidity	dry	cold
Season	spring	summer	*seasons' end	autumn	winter
Yin Organ	liver	heart	spleen	lungs	kidneys
Yang Organ	gall bladder	small intestine	stomach	large intestine	urinary bladder
Emotion	ardor	joy	worry	sadness	anxiety
Pathological Emotion	anger	overexcitement	obsession	depression	fear
Faculty	*Hun* memory	*Shen* intelligence	*Yi* reflection	*Po* instinct	*Zhi* will
Therapeutic Sound	"Shu" "Pa"	"Khe" "Haa"	"Hu" "Mei"	"Sss" "Ni"	"Chui" "Hong"
Human Sound	scream	laughter	song	weeping	sigh
Sense Organ	eyes	tongue	lips	nose	ears
Tissue	tendons, sinews	blood vessels	flesh, muscles	skin, hair	bones, teeth
Eye	iris	eye corners	eyelids	sclera	pupil
Secretion	tears	sweat	saliva	mucus	urine
Taste	acid	bitter	sweet	acrid	salty
Odor	rancid	burned	perfumed	spicy	fetid
Cereal	wheat, oats	corn, amaranth	millet, barley	rice	beans
Domestic Animal	chicken	sheep	ox	horse	pig
Planet	Jupiter	Mars	Saturn	Venus	Mercury

The last eighteen days of every season

How to Practice Qigong

Qigong has four purposes:

- To regulate the body (with dynamic exercises)
- To regulate the breath (with breathing techniques)
- To regulate the mind (with mental concentration on the circulation of energy in the meridians)
- To regulate the emotions (with emission of therapeutic sounds, the vibrations of which influence the internal organs and the nervous system)

These life-prolonging exercises are preventive and curative and exert the following effects:

- They strengthen energetic potential and spread energies evenly along the meridians.
- They improve blood circulation.
- They reinforce the immune system.
- They reestablish equilibrium in the emotions and calm the cerebral cortex, inducing serenity.
- They bring harmony to breathing and body movement.
- They increase the flexibility of the joints.
- They cure chronic disturbances.

Basic Rules

Consistency and Regularity. Practice the exercises for at least a quarter of an hour (more if possible) every day without exception. You can always find fifteen minutes, especially if you decide to change your attitude toward how you should live. It is enough to think, "I have time for myself." Do not let yourself be distracted or blocked by your family and friends; they will be grateful later when they find you decidedly more serene and expansive.

Patience and Faith. You will notice improvements after a month or two of practice, sometimes even earlier. Persevere! Set aside every doubt; the exercises are more efficacious if you do them with-

out skepticism. Do not rush; it is better to do one exercise calmly than to dash through ten in a row.

Silence and Concentration. To attain inner calm it is important to be centered in yourself. If you feel nervous, first do the exercises explained in Chapter 3 or one or two of the meridian-opening exercises in Chapter 4. Do *not* let yourself be interrupted or distracted (a "Do Not Disturb" notice on your door might be handy); do *not* answer the telephone. Choose a suitable time and a quiet, airy room and turn this daily custom into a precious moment. Before you begin, bathe and put on comfortable clothes and cotton shoes—at any rate, shoes without rubber or plastic soles, as these materials do not allow for the passage of negative ions. Distance yourself from all thoughts liable to distract you and center yourself on the rhythm of your breathing. Feel yourself rooted in the soil of the earth. If possible, practice in the open air to better absorb the cosmic and earthly energies.

Acupuncture/Moxa/Acupressure

Digital acupressure, the application of pressure by the fingers on the sensitive points of the Chinese meridians, is a gentle form of acupuncture and dates back even farther than acupuncture itself, in which needles are inserted into the skin to stimulate the same points. Even before the discovery of the meridians, the Chinese of the Neolithic age were practicing a crude form of acupressure using small, tapered stone rods, which archaeologists have discovered in tombs dating back to that distant time.

The key points of the body, the "pulse points" of health, were discovered empirically by shamans, the priests and healers of the ancient world. These shamans had observed that certain tender points under the skin invariably corresponded with certain illnesses and that by massaging the points they could alleviate not only localized discomfort but the illnesses themselves. Once they had drawn up a map of the sensitive points, these healers realized that the messages produced by pressing on each point were transmitted to the next along an invisible channel, leading finally to an internal organ, the activity of which could in this way be either stimulated or moderated.

The earliest known sketches of the meridian system were carved on the shells of turtles, creatures symbolic of longevity; these incised shells date back to the fifteenth century B.C. Eleven centuries later the foundations of acupuncture were complete, gathered together in a manual compiled at the time that China was unified by the emperor Huang Ti, whose famous mausoleum, guarded by an army of terracotta figures, is now a tourist attraction at Xi'an. This ruthless sovereign classified the work as "the emperor's classic study of internal medicine" and confined to the flames all versions predating his ascension to the throne—in particular the Confucian texts, which he found too "liberal."

At that time doctors were already using metal needles in series of differing lengths, sometimes fashioned of silver or gold—the "royal," or "noble," metals. Even today gold needles are preferred for curing infections, since gold, held to be yin, "cold," has the capacity to reduce the heat of an infection.

Once inserted in the skin so as to puncture the neuralgic meridian point (producing at times a painful reaction similar to an electric shock), the needles are manipulated and rotated in different ways, depending on whether a stimulating or calming effect is desired, an increase or dispersion of energy. The heads of the needles may also be heated, using a smoldering stick of the medicinal herb moxa.

Moxa is the Japanese name for a variety of artemisia, also called Chinese mugwort, an herb that is frequently wrapped in a thin piece of paper and rolled to create a kind of large cigar that burns very slowly. Moxa can be used even without needles to heat the acupuncture points from a distance of one centimeter from the skin. According to legend, the therapeutic use of heat was discovered by a mandarin who fell asleep on top of a rock heated by his campfire and was healed of the pain in his back.

After this it became the custom to use small sticks of blazing wood, and then in the seventh century B.C. artemisia, or moxa. Prepared packets of moxa may be found in shops selling herbs and in the Chinese quarters of many cities.

Digital acupressure (or reflexology), the massage of meridian points corresponding to all the internal organs, was discovered in a later epoch and developed into a working system at the time of the Ming emperors in the fourteenth century A.D. It forms part of the broader science of massage, which is no minor branch of Chinese medicine but a therapy practiced in hospitals often by very famous doctors and used successfully to cure even the gravest illnesses.

Cautions When Using Acupressure

In your search for the right points to press, remember that these are usually tender, even painful, under pressure, so it should not be difficult to identify them with the help of the diagrams. To locate them in relation to anatomical features, certain specific measurements are used: the *palm,* the width of your own hand across your second finger joints; and the *distance* (also known as *cun*), measured by the width of your thumb at the top thumb joint (also the length of the middle joint of the third finger). A palm is equal to three distances, or cuns (Figure 2).

In most of the meridians the points are paired and symmetrical, especially on the face, the back, and the limbs. You should massage these pairs at the same time, using both hands. Of course, when the points are located on the arms and hands, you will massage first one—the left for men and the right for women—and then the other. The special meridians are not paired but single, so you press only one point at a time on these. In this book we are dealing primarily with the Ren Mai and Du Mai, the two meridians that follow the front and back of the body's central axis.

In general, you will be using a *circular massage* with the tip of the index finger on the indicated point, continuing for about two minutes. Later, as I will explain, it will be necessary instead to *tap* the point with your finger or with a rounded rod. At other times I will ask you to *stroke* the skin with the palm of your hand, up and down.

With the help of acupressure, a large number of minor problems can be resolved easily and innocuously, without needles and without medicines that damage the body. These remedies can also be applied to children. Naturally, more complex illnesses require diagnosis from a medical doctor.

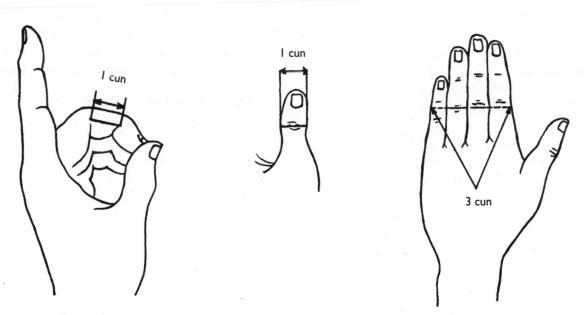

I cun = I distance

3 cun = 3 distances, a palm

Figure 2: Measurements for locating acupuncture points

1
Exuberant Vitality

Are you listless and exhausted? How can you shake off that lethargy and regain your energy quickly? Here are some fast, easy-to-do exercises you can use to help you during the course of the day.

Health at Your Fingertips

(five minutes minimum)

This first exercise is truly valuable. It serves to stimulate and balance the principal functions of the body. Practice it with regularity and you will live a long life.

You can do it anytime, anywhere—on the bus, at the movies, in front of the TV. If you suffer from insomnia, repeat it at bedtime. Do it to relax whenever you feel nervous or when you are cold or tired. Its effects on health are measureable: If your blood has been recently analyzed, repeat the analysis after three months of practice—you will see proof of improvement.

The exercise is easy: With the thumb and index finger of one hand, press the tips of the fingers of the other hand. This pressure improves the circulation of energy along the six acupuncture channels terminating in the five fingers. Tibetan monks apply a similar technique to keep their strength up in their harsh, high-altitude climate: During prayers they press the beads of a rosary between their fingers, following a fixed course. At the same time they match their breath to the rhythm of the moments of pressure by chanting a mantra.

Although this exercise may seem boring at first, it will soon win you over because you will feel *immediate* benefits—unlike the practice of most other Chinese exercises, the effects of which are felt only after a certain period of practice.

Women. Begin the exercise on the *right* hand. Press your little finger 29 times (or if you have more time and want more of a "rush," 39 or 49—up to 99 times). Then press your middle finger, and then move on to your thumb. Be sure to press each of these fingers the same number of times. Next press your ring finger and then your index finger 30 to 100 times.

Switch to the *left* hand and press, 29 to 99 times, first your thumb, then your middle finger, then your little finger. Press your index finger, then your ring finger 30 to 100 times. Be sure to press all the fingers on your left hand the same number of times you pressed the fingers on your right hand (see Figure 3).

Men. Press the fingers of each hand in the same sequence indicated for women, but start with the *left* hand (thumb, then middle finger, then little finger; index finger, then ring finger). Switch next to the *right* hand (little finger, then middle finger, then thumb; ring finger, then index finger).

Before you begin, stretch out and get comfortable. Apply pressure when you exhale, calmly and rhythmically, and release pressure when you inhale. Keep an even, natural rhythm. Count. Try to "unify mind and body," as the Chinese say. Concentrate on what you are doing. Imagine the flow of energy ris-ing from your fingertips up along your arms and into your chest. If you prefer, in order not to be distracted by random thoughts, close your eyes and as you count, mentally visualize each number. Relax. Do not give way to nervousness; do not strain. Things turn out better when you do not force them.

Begin by pressing each finger 29 or 30 times. Work your way quickly to 39 or 40 repetitions as a minimum. Go ahead and do more if you have the time and inclination. Remember: It is better to limit yourself to 29 or 30 than to skip the exercise entirely for a day. It is also better to exercise briefly twice a day than to wait for the right time for a long series.

You can teach this exercise to children. If they are too young, you can be the one to press their fingers—slowly and in this case without trying to match the pressing to the breath. Watch these children grow up strong, healthy, and robust!

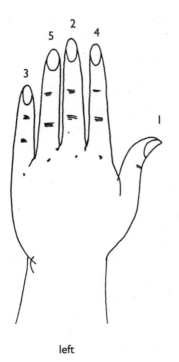

left

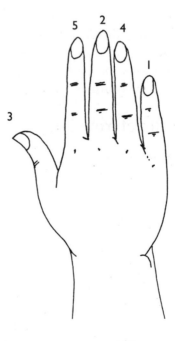

right

Figure 3: Health at your fingertips

The Nine Points of Youth

(ten minutes)

Pressing this series of nine specific acupuncture points is a lightning-quick remedy for exhaustion and nervousness. It can be done anywhere: in the office, on the bus, while watching a movie. Practiced daily, it is guaranteed to keep you in good form and to prevent a number of ailments. It is advisable to first massage each of the nine points in a circular manner and then to press them about 30 times with the tip of your finger or with the rounded point of a small rod or pencil. The points are as follows:

1. *Baihui* (20 DM): on the top of the head, where the imaginary line connecting the tips of the ears crosses (see Figure 8). *Baihui* stimulates the circulation of energy in the brain.

2. *Yintang* (1 Ext): between the eyebrows (see Figure 4). *Yintang*, one of the extra points not considered part of a meridian, is very useful in the alleviation of headaches, for which you should also pinch this point between two fingers.

3. *Renzhong* (26 DM): under the nose, halfway between the nose and the lips (see Figure 4). This is an invigorating point, useful even for fainting or sudden illness, as it restores the senses to one so affected. Pressing *Renzhong* moreover improves the sexual response in women.

These first three points stimulate the frontal meridian Ren Mai and the dorsal meridian Du Mai.

4. *Tiantu* (22 RM): in the hollow at the base of the neck, between the knobs on the collarbone (see Figure 4). *Tiantu* stimulates the thyroid and prevents asthma, coughs, and sore throats.

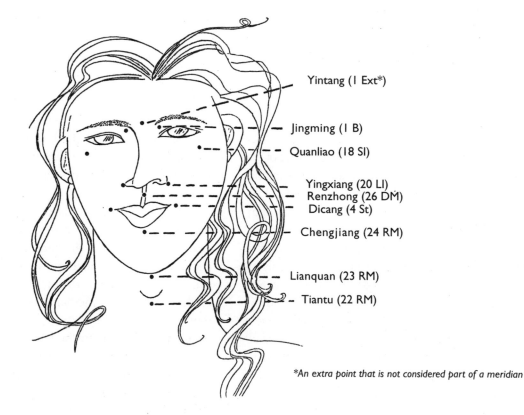

Yintang (1 Ext*)

Jingming (1 B)

Quanliao (18 SI)

Yingxiang (20 LI)
Renzhong (26 DM)
Dicang (4 St)

Chengjiang (24 RM)

Lianquan (23 RM)

Tiantu (22 RM)

An extra point that is not considered part of a meridian

Figure 4: The points of the face

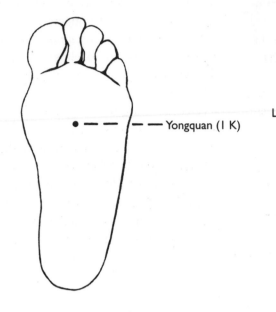

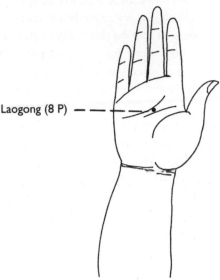

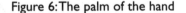

Figure 5: The sole of the foot

Figure 6: The palm of the hand

5. *Yongquan* (1 K): under the arch of the foot (see Figure 5). *Yongquan*, or "the bubbling spring of energy," is so named because of an ancient belief that the energy of the earth is absorbed by the sole of the foot at exactly this point, in the hollow of the arch. This conviction explains why Chinese masters prefer to practice in parks and gardens, where earth energy is more accessible. *Yongquan* is a notably effective point: It lowers blood pressure; alleviates tensions at the level of the lumbar vertebrae and the solar plexus; and is also efficacious in the treatment of migraines, nausea, shock, and infantile convulsions. After applying acupressure, energetically massage the sole of the foot up and down with the palm of your hand. You will feel relaxed and refreshed.

6. *Laogong* (8 P): located under the tip of the middle finger when the finger is folded down onto the palm of the hand (fold all three joints). Also known as the "palace of weariness," it calms nervous tension and reinforces the immune system (see Figure 6).

7. *Tanzhong* (17 RM): located on the sternum at the level of the nipples, it is tender when pressed (see Figure 7). This is the zone of the thymus, the gland that controls the immune system and that in China is associated with longevity. It is also, according to Chinese medicine, the center of emotion. With your closed fist, gently beat the zone running down along the sternum, from the base of the neck to the point *Tanzhong,* as in mea culpa, mea culpa. This exercise calms asthma and stimulates the lungs and bronchi. It also reduces anxiety; try it when some emotion or fear makes you feel that "your heart is in your throat."

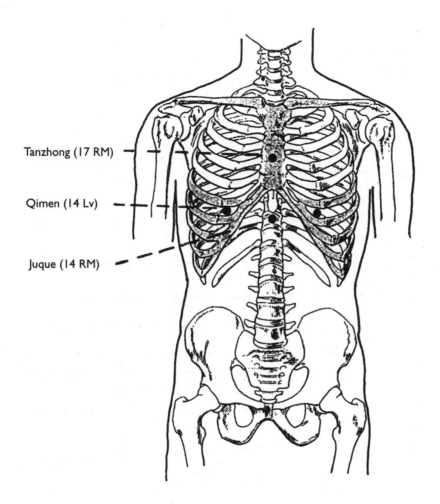

Tanzhong (17 RM)

Qimen (14 Lv)

Juque (14 RM)

Figure 7: Some points around the sternum

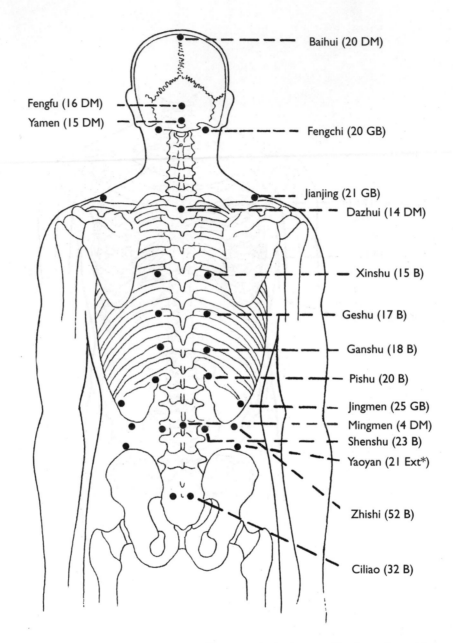

Baihui (20 DM)

Fengfu (16 DM)
Yamen (15 DM)

Fengchi (20 GB)

Jianjing (21 GB)
Dazhui (14 DM)

Xinshu (15 B)

Geshu (17 B)

Ganshu (18 B)

Pishu (20 B)

Jingmen (25 GB)
Mingmen (4 DM)
Shenshu (23 B)
Yaoyan (21 Ext*)

Zhishi (52 B)

Ciliao (32 B)

*An extra point that is not considered part of a meridian

Figure 8: Some points on the back

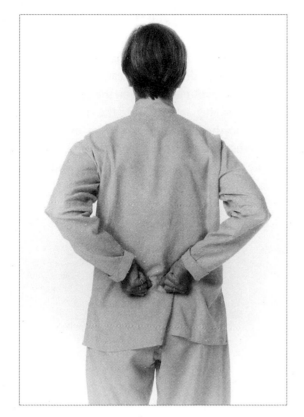

Photo 1

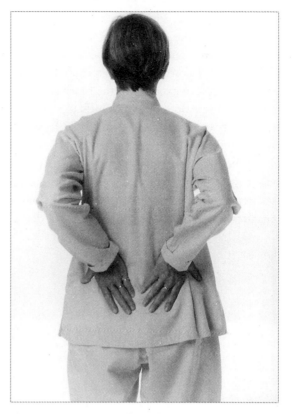

Photo 2

8. *Mingmen* (4 DM): is known as the "door of life" (see Photos 1 and 2). It is located on the vertebral column at the level of the second lumbar vertebra at the waist (see Figure 8). To stimulate this point, massage it with closed fists in the following manner: Charge your fists with energy by rubbing them one against the other; then, leaning slightly forward, thump them along two parallel lines about two fingers distant from the spine, drumming all the lower zone of the back, up and down, above and below the *Mingmen* point. Then do the same on the sacral bone. To finish, heat the palms of your hands by rubbing them one against the other and then vigorously massage the area of the two kidneys up and down for about three minutes.

Your kidneys are filters. If too many toxins are circulating in your body, the kidneys cannot eliminate all the waste material, which then accumulates and gives rise to obstructions, high blood pressure, and kidney stones. Drumming with the fists on this area loosens the sediments and aids their elimination. This exercise is also useful for other problems: irregular menstruation, lumbago, sciatica, hemorrhoids, chronic fatigue, and impotence in men. According to Taoist medicine, the kidneys are the receptacles of the precious qi, especially sexual energy, and are therefore the "door of life." The sacrum is also important because it is connected, by way of the spinal cord, to the brain.

9. The *dantian:* is known as "field of cinnabar" and is located at the center of the lower abdomen, between the navel and the pubic bone (see Figure 9 and Photo 3). According to Taoist tradition, this is the area strategic to excellence, the place where qi is stored. Rub the palms of your hands together until they heat up and then place them (right hand first, covered by the left for women; left hand first, covered by the right for men) on your stomach below the rib cage. Massage the whole abdomen in a clockwise circular motion, gradually descending from the stomach to the lower abdomen, or groin. The dantian zone should be massaged in this clockwise direction about 30 times. This is helpful in cases of constipation; to alleviate diarrhea, massage the area in a counterclockwise direction instead.

Concentrate your attention on the various organs you are massaging and visualize the energy you are spreading to them. This massage is a miracle cure for many disturbances. It regulates the intestines and stimulates the liver, stomach, appetite, and digestion, as well as improving hormone production.

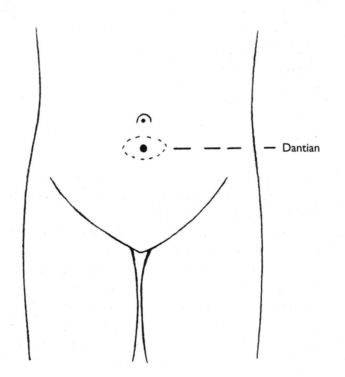

Figure 9: The dantian

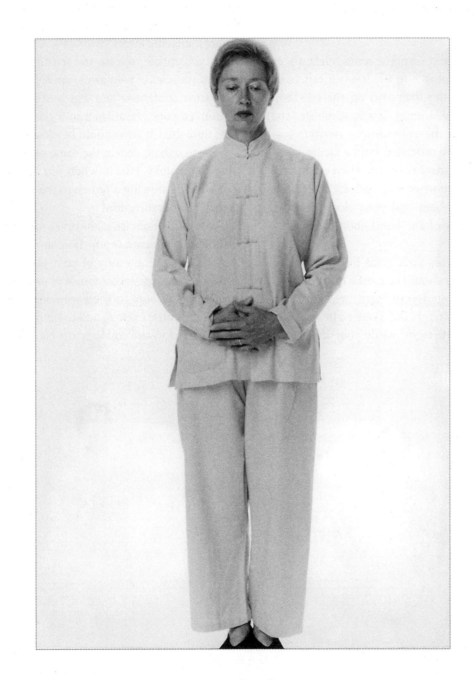

Photo 3

"Launching the Fists with a Fierce Glance"

(eight minutes)

This is the seventh exercise in the series "eight pieces of brocade" (see Photos 4 to 8). It has a beneficial effect on the qi of the liver and on the eyes and muscles, which it invigorates. It also stimulates the cerebral cortex and the autonomous nervous system. It is particularly indicated before facing situations of conflict or to restore energy when exhausted.

Assume the position of a horseback rider with your knees sharply bent and your closed fists on your hips (the back of the hand should be facing earthward).

As you inhale, cross your arms in front of your chest (your right arm should be closest to your body) while you straighten out your legs.

As you exhale, stretch out your right arm and throw a punch to the right, while your left fist re-turns to its original position high on the left hip. At the same time, bend your legs as far as you can, turn your head to the left, and gaze in that direction with fierce, menacing eyes.

As you inhale, release the tension in your eyes and the muscles of your arms, open your fists, lower both arms, straighten your legs, and cross your arms in front of your chest again in a gentle movement. This time the left arm should be closest to the body.

As you exhale, repeat the same sequence of motions to the right. That is, when you flex your knees, you will be throwing a punch to the left and gazing fiercely in that direction.

Repeat this exercise eight times for each side.

Focus. Concentrate on the contraction of your muscles and the intensity of your glance while you exhale and on the relaxation of your muscles while you inhale. Be sure to keep your shoulders relaxed during the entire exercise and to tilt the pelvis to aim the tailbone forward and keep the back from arching.

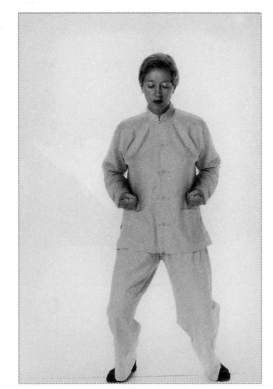

Photo 4

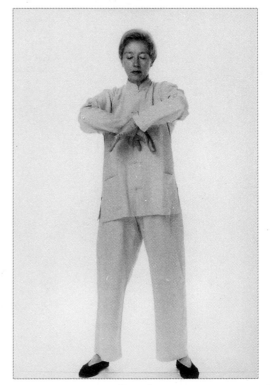

Photo 5

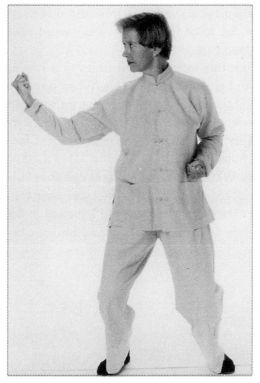

Photo 6

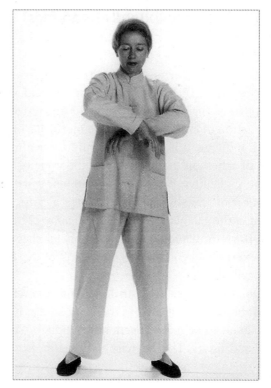

Photo 7

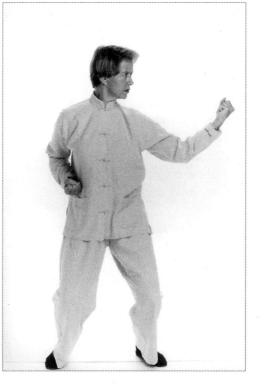

Photo 8

"The Eagle Extends Its Wings"

(five minutes)

This is the fifth exercise in the Wudang series (see Photos 9 to 13). It opens both the yin and yang energies of the arms and brings harmony to the circulation of energy between the meridians of the arms and legs. It is also wonderful for the alleviation of aches and pains in the shoulder joints. It is notably effective in combating fatigue, since the rotation of the shoulders stimulates a particular point of the gall bladder meridian, *Jianjing* (21 GB), and this stimulation exerts a beneficial effect on the energy currents in the meridians of the liver and gall bladder.

One of the liver's various functions is to render fluid the movement of qi in the body, so that it can flow freely to help the spleen, heart, kidneys, stomach, and lungs. This exercise is therefore particularly useful when the qi of the liver is blocked by the emotions.

While inhaling, take a step forward with your left foot, shifting the weight of your body onto your bent left leg. At the same time, raise your outstretched left arm, with the palm of your hand facing up, in the direction of your left foot and bring it all the way up to a vertical position above your head. At this point, as you exhale, shift the weight of your body onto your bent right leg and lower your left arm, palm of the hand facing down, behind you, turning your head to follow the motion with your gaze. At the same time, begin to raise your right arm (with the palm of the hand facing up), so that your arms form a straight line.

Shift your weight forward onto your left foot again as you raise your right arm over your head. As you exhale, shift the weight onto your bent right leg and lower your right arm, palm of the hand facing down, behind you, while you raise your left arm, with the palm of the hand facing up, until your arms form a straight line. Only the movement of the left arm, when your step forward has been on the left, and of the right arm, when your step forward has been on the right, are to be followed by your turned head and directed gaze.

Perform this rotation eight times in a row as loosely and gracefully as possible. When you have completed the eighth rotation, repeat the same series of movements on the right, starting this time by taking a step forward with the right foot and proceeding from there.

Focus. While inhaling, concentrate on your little finger and then on your thumb; while exhaling, concentrate on the point *Laogong* (8 P), located in the center of the palm of the hand you are lowering behind you.

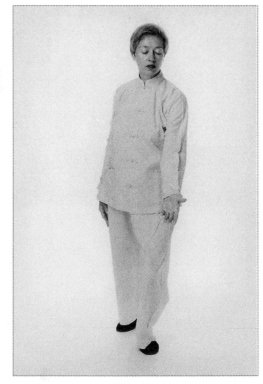

Photo 9

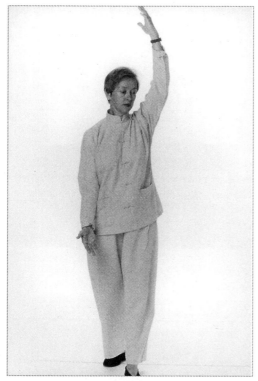

Photo 10

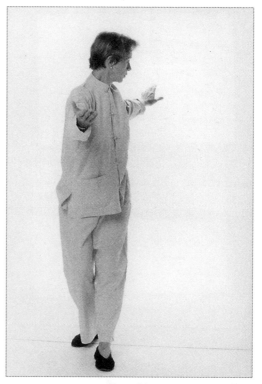

Photo 11

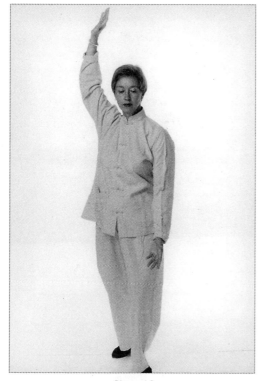

Photo 12

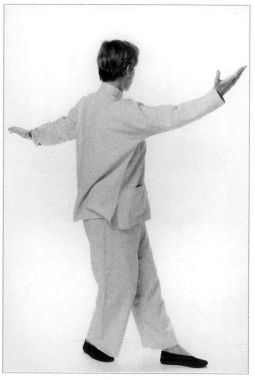

Photo 13

2
Beautiful and Slim

Healthy = beautiful, beautiful = healthy: Practitioners of traditional Chinese medicine make no distinction between aesthetics and health. They know how to improve a patient's outer aspect by reestablishing energetic equilibrium in the internal organs and, vice versa, how to ameliorate the patient's health by means of effective aesthetic treatments. When they wish to make wrinkles, age spots, bags under the eyes, or slack muscles disappear, they act on the meridians that link skin, eyes, and muscles to the internal source of their problems—that is, they work on both the symptom and its cause. So do not be surprised when I suggest that you use these "beauty" exercises to resolve other, more serious, problems as well. The first exercise we deal with here, for example, tones facial muscles and prevents wrinkles but also, by stimulating the many meridians underlying the face, improves both sight and hearing and alleviates headaches. Traditional Chinese doctors interest themselves in our morale, as well: They advise us to stay calm for the sake of our figures and help us to redis-cover serenity with their exercises for good health and beauty, accompanied by massage and breathing techniques, mental concentration, and autosuggestion to relax and expand the nerves and mind.

Each of the following massages and exercises should be done at least 10 times in a row. The points should be pressed, or better yet massaged, with a circular motion.

Qigong Against Wrinkles: Massaging the Face

Here is a quick exercise that can be practiced whenever you feel tired, wherever you are and at any time of the day.

With the tip of your tongue resting against your palate, inhale deeply while rubbing the palms of your hands together for about a minute or until they feel warm.

Press your palms against your closed eyes for 10 seconds or so, exhaling and focusing on the energy and warmth penetrating your eyes. Then, with your hands resting on either side of your nose, lightly massage your face outward from the nose to the ears, imagining that your skin is becoming ever smoother. According to the doctor who taught me these exercises—Grace Yu, a woman from Shanghai who is sixty years old and looks forty—it is crucially important to convince oneself of the efficacy of the treatment.

Next, stroke your face, massaging it with your palms from the chin to the roots of the hair, your two middle fingers working up the sides of the nose. When your fingertips touch your hair, separate your hands and massage along the hairline down over the temples, in front of the ears, and along the jaw. By the time you reach your chin again, you will have massaged the entire outer perimeter of your face.

Repeat this massage 18 times. It will activate blood circulation, balance the functions of the sebaceous glands, and improve the metabolism of the cells. The efficacy of the exercise becomes even greater if, like the Chinese, you mentally evoke the path of the vital energy qi, which originates in the dantian zone (in the center of the abdomen, three fingers' width below the navel, inside the womb—see Figure 9) and rises up along the median part of the torso to the collarbone, where it branches off to flow down the arms until it reaches the center of the hands. With regular practice you will feel a pleasant sensation of warmth.

Forehead. With your index and middle fingers joined on both hands, massage upward along the middle of your forehead, from the point *Yintang* (1 Ext, see Figure 4) to your hairline. Next massage outward from the center of your forehead toward your temples, moving along the eyebrows. Finally massage the point *Taiyang* (3 Ext, see Figure 10), located at the outer tip of the eyebrows in the hollow of the temple. Do this nine times, working circularly and moving backward toward the hairline. This massage is also useful for headaches and weariness.

Nose. Rub up and down the sides of your nose, using your index fingers. This is useful for preventing or attenuating the wrinkles that form on either side of your nose, as well as for curing colds and bouts of sinusitis. Massage the *Yingxiang* points toward the outside (20 LI, at the sides of the nostrils—see Figure 4).

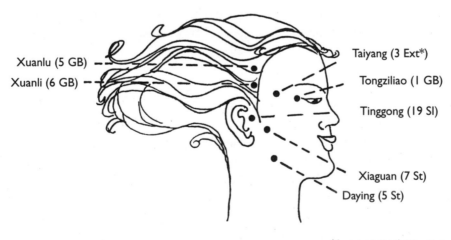

Xuanlu (5 GB)
Xuanli (6 GB)
Taiyang (3 Ext*)
Tongziliao (1 GB)
Tinggong (19 SI)
Xiaguan (7 St)
Daying (5 St)

An extra point that is not considered part of a meridian

Figure 10: The points of the face (profile)

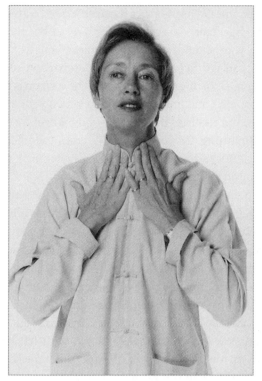

Photo 14

corners of the mouth, and eliminate wrinkles and pimples around the lips.

Neck. Strategic not only to beauty but above all to health, the neck is the passageway for eight important meridians as well as for blood vessels and nerves. Tension is manifested strongly here, whether arising from tiredness or emotional imbalance (according to traditional Chinese practitioners, emotions such as anger, fear, and sorrow correspond to energy blocks in the organs they influence and by which they are influenced). When tension accumulates in the neck, its muscles rigidify and reduce blood flow to the brain. The importance of keeping the neck relaxed becomes obvious, then, both for unimpeded circulation and for the prevention or alleviation of bad moods.

Massage your neck with the palms of your hands, from the collarbone up, 36 times (Photo 14). Smile beautifully while visualizing that you are smoothing and polishing your skin. Then massage downward from the chin to the base of the neck, alternating hands, 36 times. This massage stimulates the thyroid and the whole metabolism and is helpful in losing weight.

Other Techniques for Toning the Skin (and the Lungs)

You can complete your face massage by going on to massage the meridians in your arms (see Chapter 4). To revitalize the lung meridian, the energy of which governs the skin, arm massage is a must (the lung meridian runs down the inside of your arms). Eventually you can add the exercises that open the meridians of the lungs and the large intestine (see Chapter 4).

The Therapeutic Sounds "Ssss" and "Ni"

In cases of chronic weakness of the lungs (sinusitis, catarrh, colds, asthma, or bronchitis) it is advisable to use sound therapy, as the Chinese have done for more than two thousand years. The relationship between the utterance of sounds, including song, and the health of the skin is based on the Chinese

Chin. Grasp your chin between your thumb and your middle finger and squeeze it 20 times. Your thumb should be positioned in the hollow above the Adam's apple (point *Lianquan,* 23 RM) and your middle finger just above the dimple in the middle of your chin (point *Chengjiang,* 24 RM—see Figure 4). This exercise tones the muscles of the neck, prevents wrinkles on the neck and lower lip, and eliminates double chin and acne.

Cheeks. Using your index, middle, and ring fingers in separate positions, press the three following points in sequence: *Xiaguan* (7 St, just in front of the tragus of the ear, in the hollow that forms there when you open your mouth—see Figure 10); *Quanliao* (18 SI, beneath the outer corner of the eye, in the hollow under the cheekbone—see Figure 4); and *Dicang* (4 St, near the corner of the lips where they join—see Figure 4).

Press these points simultaneously 20 times in a row to tone facial muscles, prevent drooping at the medicinal principle that the lungs govern the skin and are responsible for its hydration and tone.

You can either stand up or sit down for this exercise. With your arms crossed and the palms of your hands resting on your breast, inhale first, then utter the sound while you exhale, making sure that the sound vibrates all through the rib cage.

The sound "Ssss" should be gently hissed through the teeth, whereas the sound "Ni" should be pronounced forcefully during the entire length of the exhalation. These two sounds harmonize energetic circulation in the lungs and in the whole body. They also exert a calming effect on the mind and nervous system.

The voice in general is particularly linked to the energetic situation of the lungs. Weakness of the voice indicates that the energy in the lungs is operating at a deficit, and this condition of weakness—especially if it is pronounced—may manifest as lowered, whispering speech or even loss of voice.

The vocal exercises mentioned above serve to tone and strengthen the voice and are particularly useful to people in professions that strain it, such as teachers or performers. Singing is also a fine vocal exercise.

Slimming Down with the Dragon Exercises

"The Dragon Slithers up the Column"

In addition to reducing your waist size, this exercise (see Photos 15 to 19) helps relieve lumbar and shoulder pains and herniated discs. It also strengthens the blood and immune system; if you practice it for a few days, depleted blood will rise back to its normal level. It is particularly indicated for facilitating the opening of the *Mingmen* point (4 DM, see Figure 8) and easing the passage of qi across this key point, located at the level of the *second* lumbar vertebra. This exercise also helps in recovering from weakness and weariness in convalescence and is indicated for people who are ill with cancer. Paired with the practice of the therapeutic sound "Chui," it compensates for the damaging effects of chemotherapy.

Assume the position of a horseback rider, with your legs wide apart (so that your feet are set out further than your shoulders) and your knees bent as far as they can go. Keep in mind the comparison to the dragon "slithering up the column": The column is your trunk, erect and immobile, around which your arms, loose and elastic as the dragon's body, wheel.

Breathing. As you inhale, fill your abdomen so that it sticks out; when you exhale, contract your abdominal muscles.

Begin by inhaling with your hands crossed on the dantian. While you exhale, rotate your arms around your upper body, twisting your waist while your legs remain bent and solidly anchored to the ground. Follow the movement of your arms by turning your upper body, first to the left; your eyes should follow the right palm, which comes to rest on the left shoulder near the cheek. At the same time, your left arm bends low and to the back, so that your left hand ends up touching the right ribs just under the shoulder blade. Keep this position and inhale again.

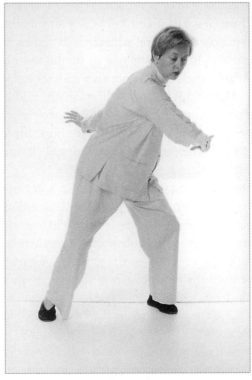

Photo 15

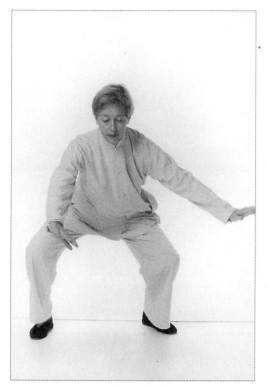

Photo 16

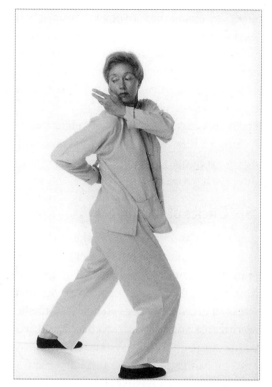

Photo 17

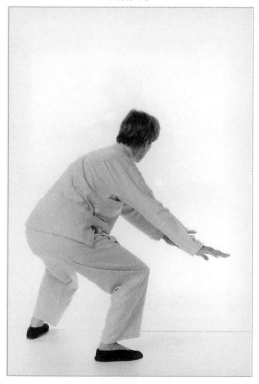

Photo 18

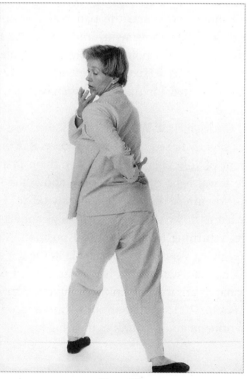

Photo 19

Exhale, reversing the movement: Your right hand rotates downward with the palm facing down, then bends behind you, coming to rest on the left ribs under the left shoulder blade, while your left palm comes to rest on your right shoulder. Keep this position and inhale again.

Repeat this exercise very slowly eight times in a row, concentrating on the point *Mingmen* and following the palm of the hand that moves toward your shoulder with your eyes.

The Six Circles of the Dragon

Are you listless and exhausted? Take on the movements of the dragon and you will feel the energy rise up renewed in your body! This ancient Taoist practice not only engages you in very effective slimming exercises but greatly increases energetic nourishment to the three cavities (lungs, stomach, and womb) and to the entire endocrine system. In fact, it stimulates the pineal gland and the pituitary gland (first movement), the suprarenal and genital glands (second movement), the suprarenal and thymus glands (third movement), and the pancreas and spleen (fourth and fifth movement) and opens the solar plexus and the *Shu* points, "doors" to the internal organs, on the back (sixth movement). The exercise is also indicated for diabetes, hypoglycemia, and lumbago.

1. *Circle on High:* With your feet joined and your knees slightly flexed, join your hands as if in prayer in front of your solar plexus. Move them in a half circle toward the right and rising above the head while you inhale deeply. Then as you exhale, bring your hands down to the left until they complete the circle, returning to their original position. Meanwhile, swing your knees to the side in the direction opposite your hands; that is, toward the left when your hands are rotating on the right and vice versa (see Photos 20 to 25). Your body should move in a serpentine manner—think of the dragon.

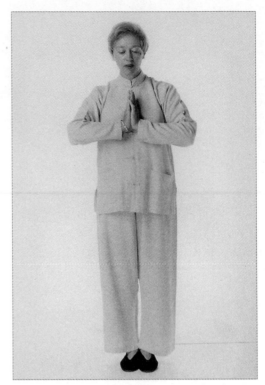

Photo 20

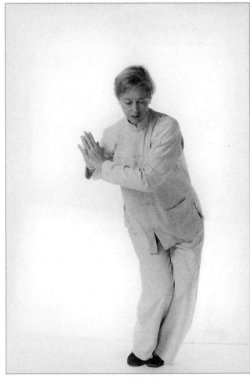

Photo 21

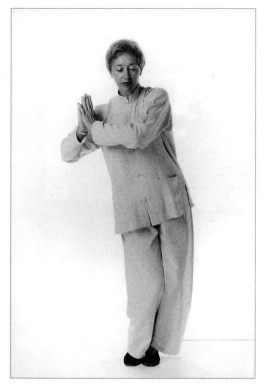

Photo 22

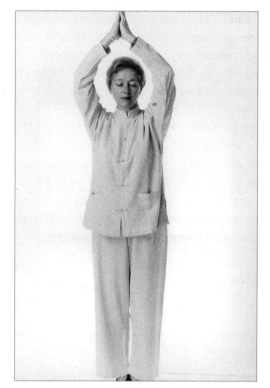

Photo 23

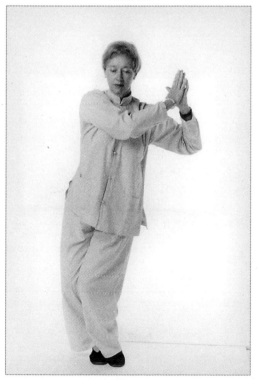

Photo 24

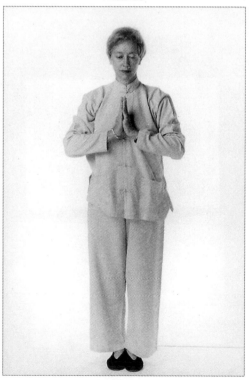

Photo 25

2. *Circle Low:* Start from the same position as in the exercise above. Your joined hands descend to the right and as you bend your waist describe a circle almost to your feet; then they rise to the left. As in the exercise above, swing your knees in the opposite direction. Breathe as in the exercise above (see Photos 26 to 28).

3. *Circle in Front:* Starting from the solar plexus and bending your waist forward, bring your joined hands to the right, then let them describe a wide horizontal circle. Inhale during the first half circle, exhale during the second. Be sure to keep your legs straight (see Photos 29 to 32).

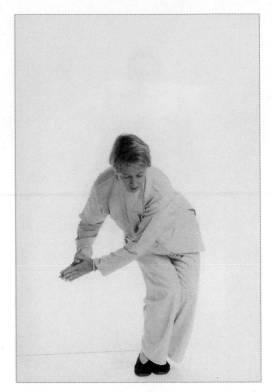

Photo 26

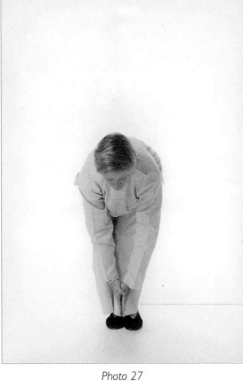

Photo 27

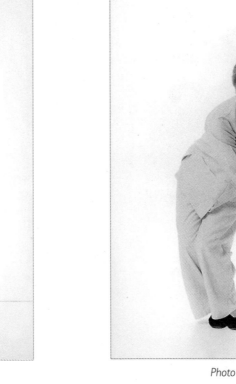

Photo 28

Beautiful and Slim

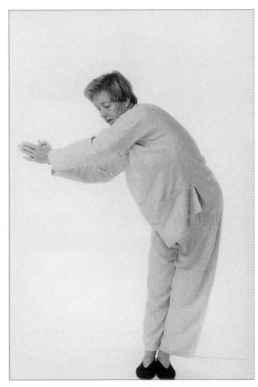

Photo 29

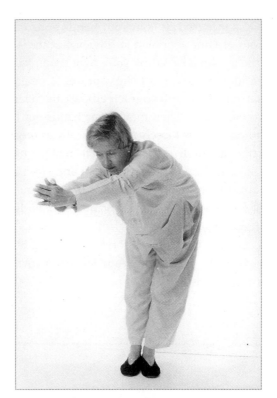

Photo 30

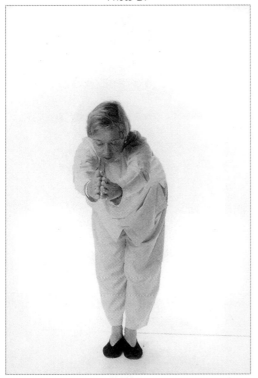

Photo 31

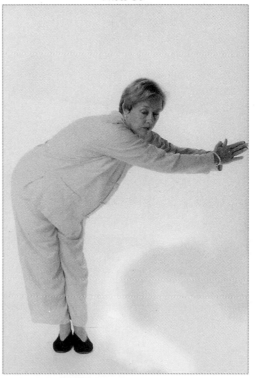

Photo 32

4. *Circle to the Left:* Join your hands horizontally in front of your abdomen at the level of the waist, your left palm covered by your right palm. Sliding the inside of your wrists along your waist, bring your hands to the left until your left elbow can no longer move backward. Then move your hands out from your body and as loosely and elastically as possible describe an ample circle to the left, making use of the "spring effect" of the first twist to bring the hands back in front of the body and return to the starting point (see Photos 33 to 37). Breathe as you did in the preceding exercises.

5. *Circle to the Right:* Perform the exercise above moving to the right, with your left palm covering your right palm.

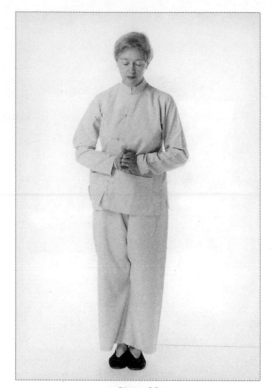

Photo 33

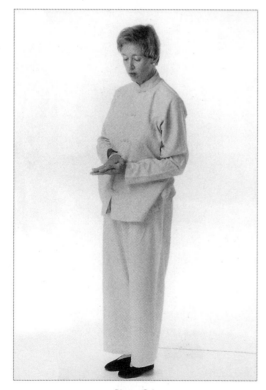

Photo 34

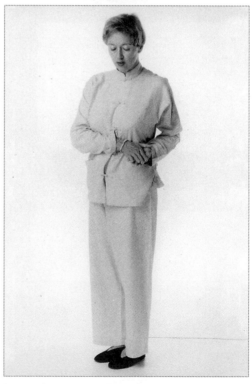

Photo 35

Beautiful and Slim

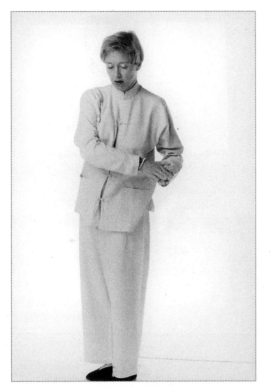

Photo 36

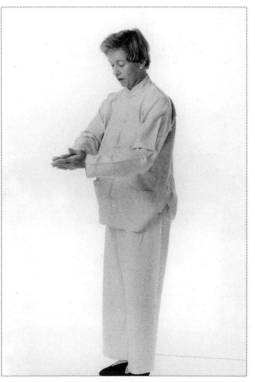

Photo 37

6. *The Salute:* Join your hands in front of the solar plexus, raise them together above your head, and straighten your arms completely as you inhale. Then as you exhale, let your arms and hands describe a large vertical circle to the front of your body, right down to your feet as you bend your waist, and bring them back to the starting point in front of your solar plexus (see Photos 38 to 44).

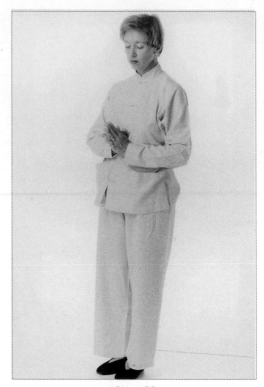

Photo 38

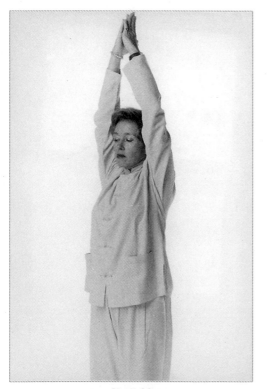

Photo 39

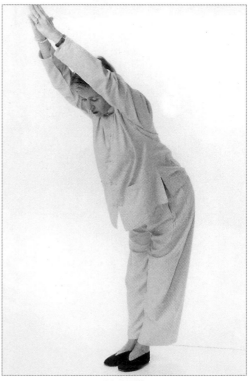

Photo 40

Beautiful and Slim

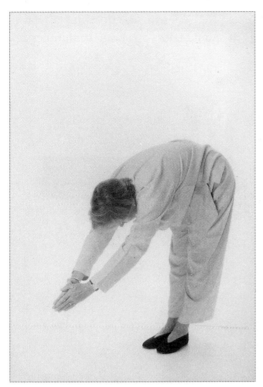

Photo 41

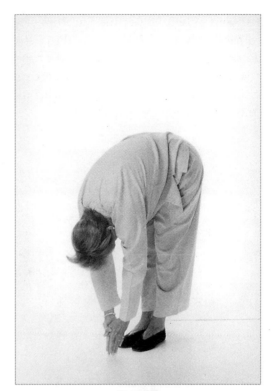

Photo 42

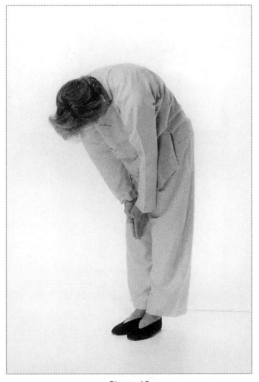

Photo 43

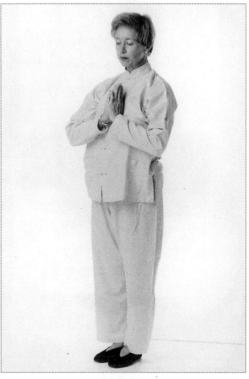

Photo 44

For your closure, lower the fingertips of your joined hands toward your abdomen; then rest your hands, with the left hand placed over the right, on your dantian. As you do this, take a slow, deep inhalation and exhalation and visualize bringing energy into this area (see Photos 45 and 46).

Repeat the series of six circles for a total of six series. It should take you about 10 minutes in all.

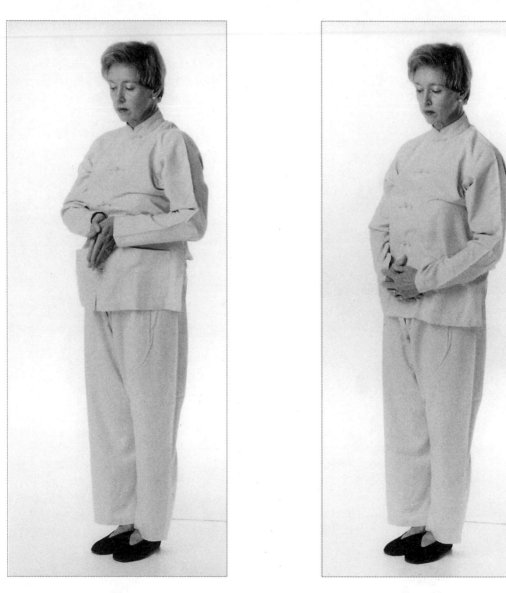

Photo 45   Photo 46

Beautiful and Slim

The Dance of the Dragon

The principle is the same as for the preceding exercise. With joined hands, describe three superimposed circles (see Photos 47 to 64): the first around the head as you rise up on the tips of your toes, the second in front of the breast, and the third in front of the lower abdomen. Be sure to draw the circles as amply and widely as possible and to always swing your knees in the direction opposite to your arms so as to emphasize the flexing movement of the spine. At the end of the exercise, raise your joined hands over your head again, then lower them to the level of the sternum for a few seconds, and finally fold them over the dantian, just below the navel, with the left hand over the right.

This exercise, performed for 10 minutes every day for two or three months, will trim you down (without your having to diet) and renew your natural beauty. It stimulates and regularizes the endocrine system and the production of hormones and tones the skin and muscles. It encourages a true, natural lymphatic drainage throughout the body conducive to the elimination of liquids and wastes. It also improves the functions of the intestines and stomach. The spine becomes looser and more flexible, benefiting the intervertebral discs. The dance of the dragon improves blood circulation as well and after a few weeks of regular practice, the skin becomes rosier and smoother.

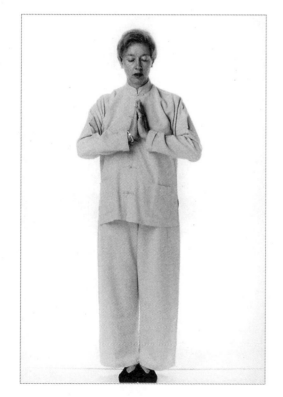

Photo 47

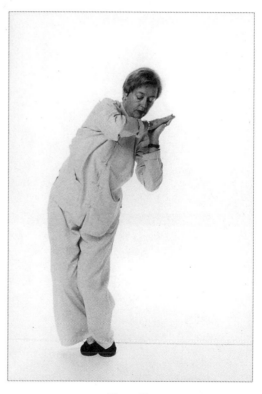

Photo 48

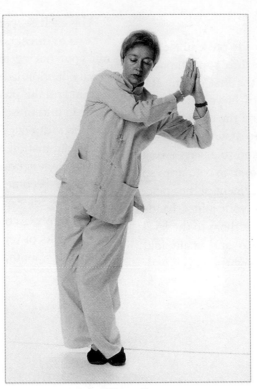

Photo 49

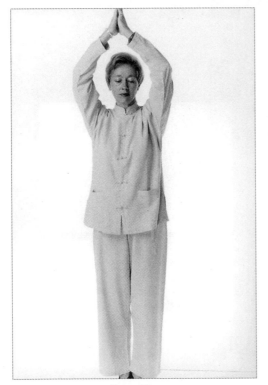

Photo 50

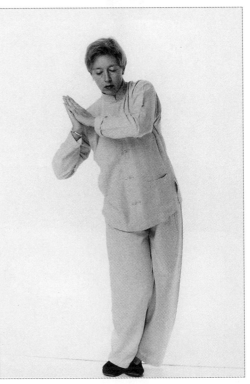

Photo 51

Beautiful and Slim

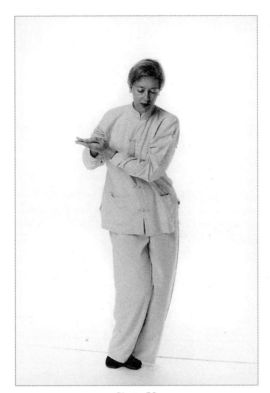

Photo 52

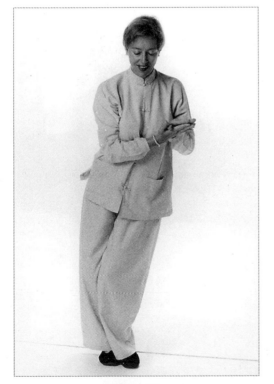

Photo 53

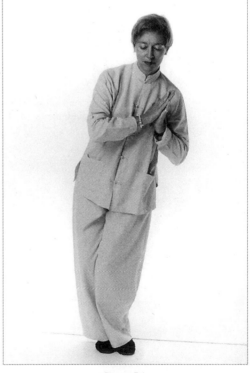

Photo 54

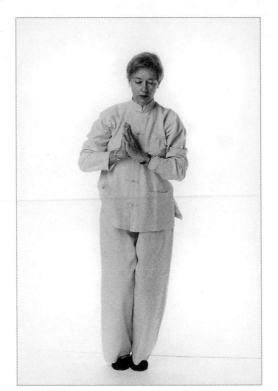

Photo 55

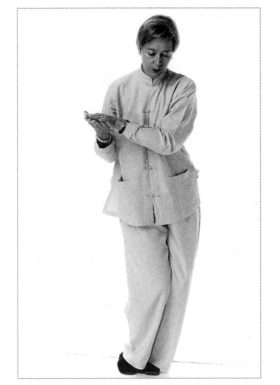

Photo 56

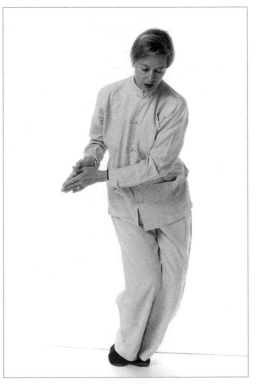

Photo 57

Beautiful and Slim

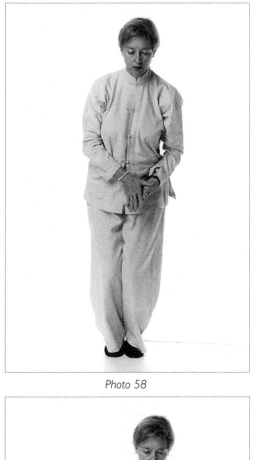

Photo 58

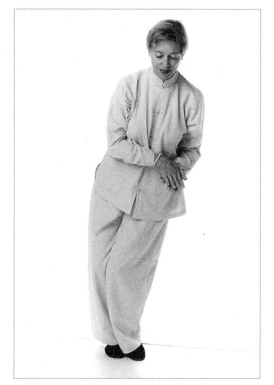

Photo 59

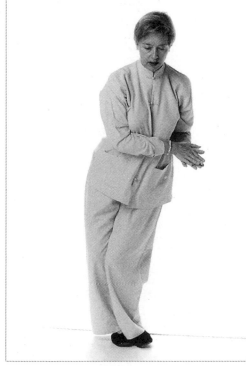

Photo 60

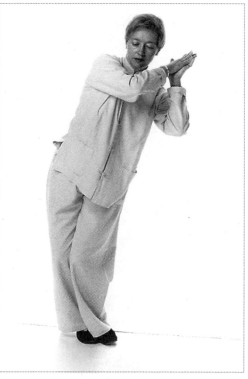

Photo 61

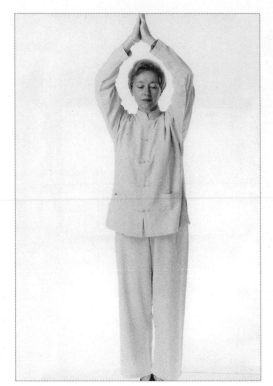

Photo 62

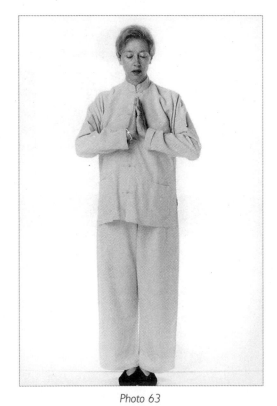

Photo 63

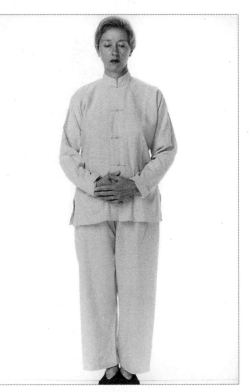

Photo 64

Exercises for the Abdominal Muscles and the Waist

1. *The Bellows* (see Photo 65): This exercise stimulates the liver and the spleen. It is particularly beneficial to smokers and to anyone who lives in a city, since it allows the alveoli of the lungs to expel toxins. Its contractions of the abdominal wall strengthen the diaphragm and the abdominal muscles, helping to reduce excess fat as well as providing a therapeutic massage of the internal organs. The "bellows" refreshes the brain, irrigating it with oxygen-rich blood. During the exercise the rhythm and volume of blood circulation rise, although the blood pressure remains level. Try this exercise when you are feeling exhausted and see how quickly you are back on your feet.

Sitting down with your legs stretched straight in front of you, bend forward and grasp the big toe on each foot between your forefinger and thumb, placing the thumb on the initial points of the two meridians of the liver and the spleen, the *Dadun* and *Yinbai* points (see Figure 12 for location of the points). If you cannot manage to reach your feet, you can grasp the backs of your ankles, calves, or knees, in which case the exercise will primarily stimulate the meridians of the bladder, lungs, and large intestine.

Bend your head forward and bring it as close as possible to your knees. Keep your elbows bent downward; your tongue should rest against your upper palate. In this position you will breathe the "bellows," seeking to expel, as forcefully as possible, all the air that is stagnating in the lungs.

To start, take a half breath, filling the lungs only halfway; then, by vigorously contracting the muscles of the abdominal wall, expel all the air from your nostrils, blowing strongly during the entire exhalation. You should be making a sound much like a strong nose-blowing—the sound of a bellows reviving the fire.

Now relax the tension in your abdomen, inhale halfway again, and repeat the exercise (about 20 breaths a minute) for two to three minutes. Take care to pause and breathe deeply in and out whenever you are left feeling breathless. The "bellows" is very powerful, so proceed gradually and without straining yourself. This rule holds true for all the exercises.

2. *The Upright Turtle* (see Photos 66 to 73): This exercise stimulates the thyroid and resolves problems of gas and indigestion. The sound that is used, "Xu," has a calming effect on the liver and gall bladder and therefore helps to dissolve impatience and anger, two negative emotions tied to these organs.

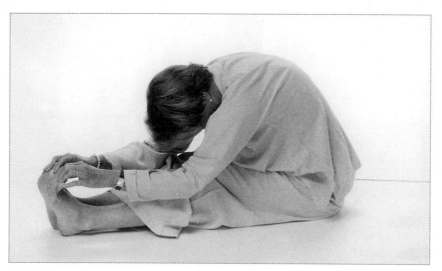

Photo 65

Stand erect with your legs straight and slightly apart, your feet in line with your hips.

While inhaling, fold your hands over the dantian, below the navel, with your right hand under your left hand for women, and your left hand under your right hand for men.

While exhaling very slowly, lean forward with your chin thrust out, bending your body only at the waist and keeping your legs straight, until your unbent torso is held parallel to the ground at right angles to your legs.

During the entire exhalation, pronounce the sound "Xu," making it last as long as possible, and press your belly with your hands to push out all the air. Maintain this position for a few seconds while easing up on your hands' pressure and letting your body relax with your head hanging down and your back slightly curved.

Now slowly straighten your back, vertebra by vertebra, while inhaling naturally, letting your diaphragm work by itself without forcing the inhalation, until you return to your initial position.

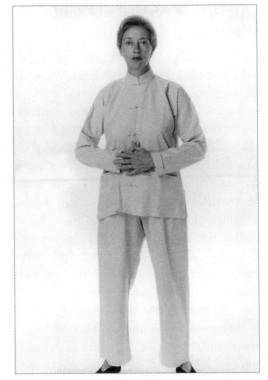

Photo 66

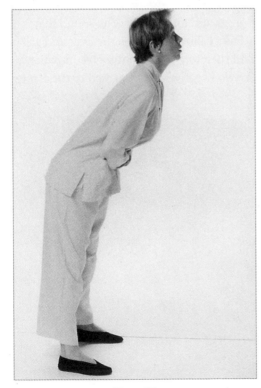

Photo 67

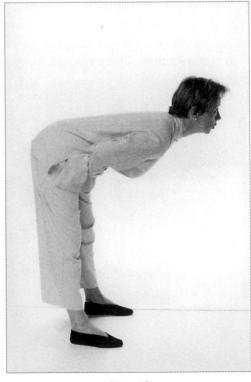

Photo 68

Beautiful and Slim

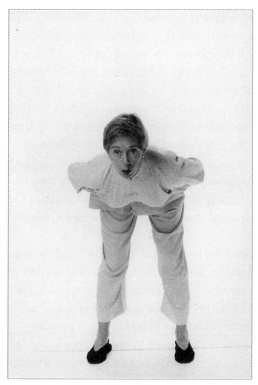

Photo 69

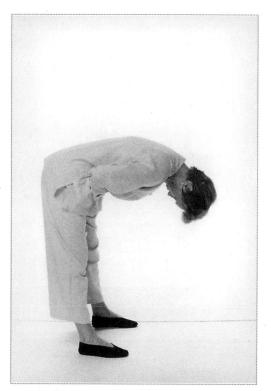

Photo 70

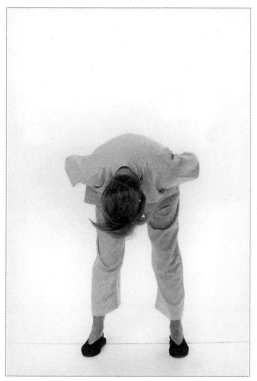

Photo 71

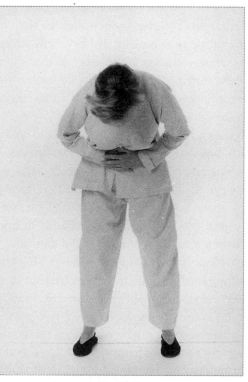

Photo 72

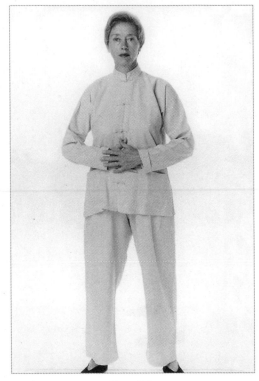

Photo 73

your shoulders against the wall. Exhaling through your mouth, push out your abdomen for the duration of the exhalation. Repeat at least 12 times.

• *Second Phase* (see Photos 74 to 77): Stand away from the wall and lift yourself up on tiptoes with your arms raised in front of your chest at the level of the shoulders. Contracting your abdominal muscles, bend your knees so that your heels are as perpendicular as possible to the floor. Try to hold this position for a few seconds, lengthening the duration gradually as you continue to practice the exercise until you can hold it for three minutes or more.

This exercise tones all the muscles of the legs and strengthens the ankles and back. The second phase also stimulates the meridians of the legs: bladder, gall bladder, and stomach, reducing retention of water and excess fat, as well as lowering blood pressure.

The two phases are complementary and should be practiced daily without exception for a minimum of two months.

Repeat this cycle twice; then after the third exhalation, inhale intentionally and forcefully while lifting your curved arms to the sides up to the level of the ears, turning the palms of your hands upward with the fingers to the outside, as if you were raising up heavy trays.

At the end of the inhalation, pause and hold your breath, without straining, for a few moments, with your back arched slightly, your shoulders raised, and your head thrown back, so that you are gazing directly above you. Then exhale while pronouncing the sound "Xu" and lower your hands in front of you to rest folded once more on the dantian.

3. *Accelerated Dantian Breathing:* This simple breathing exercise tones the abdominal muscles and quickly rids the body of excess fat and water accumulated in the tissues. It unfolds in two phases.

• *First Phase:* Standing very straight, position yourself against a wall, so that your head, back, buttocks, heels, and arms are pressed against it. Inhaling through your nose, push out your chest and press

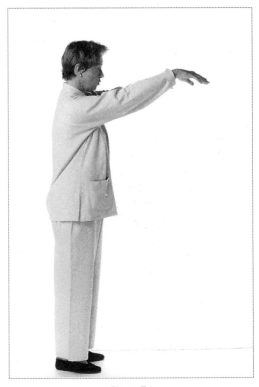

Photo 74

Beautiful and Slim

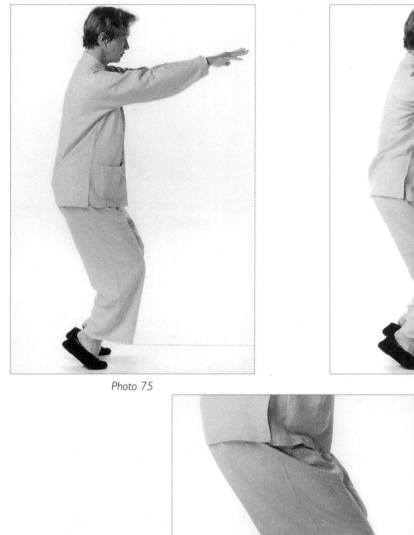

Photo 75

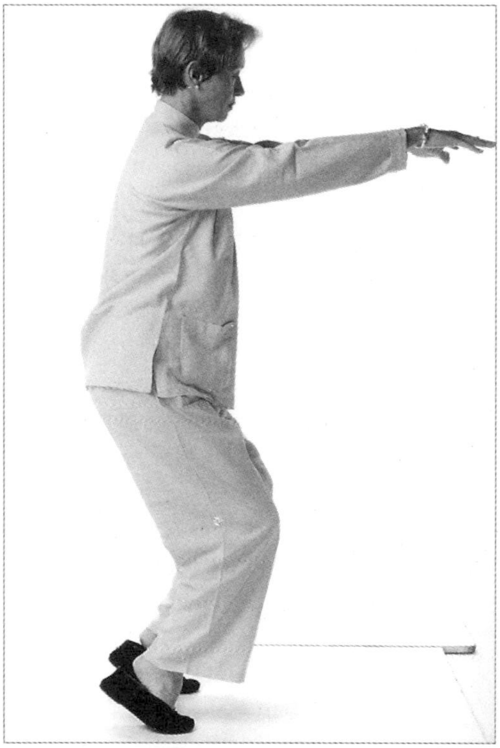

Photo 76

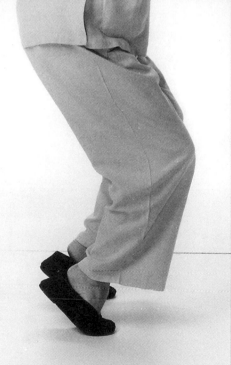

Photo 77

4. *The Cry of the Phoenix in the Sky* (see Photos 78 to 84): Start from an erect position. Raise your outstretched right arm above your head and, bending forward, lower and rotate your arm toward your left foot while lifting your left arm behind your back.

Now place the back of your right hand on the outside edge of your left foot; turn the palm inward and let it slide upward along the outside of the left leg until it reaches your waist.

Straighten your torso with your arms outstretched to either side at the level of the shoulders, then repeat the entire movement, this time to the right, raising your left arm above your head and lowering it toward the right foot.

This exercise slims the waist and makes it more flexible. It also relieves lumbar aches and pains. Repeat it a minimum of eight times.

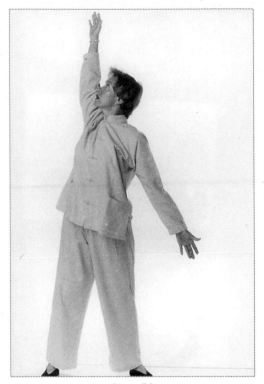

Photo 78

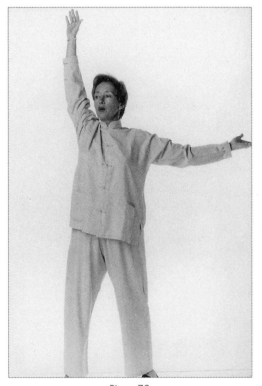

Photo 79

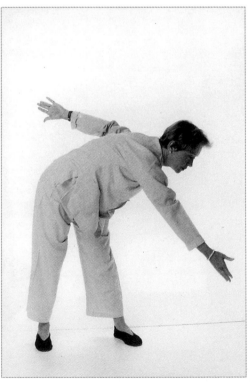

Photo 80

Beautiful and Slim

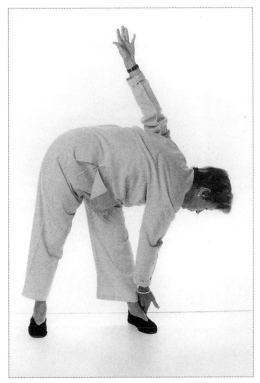

Photo 81

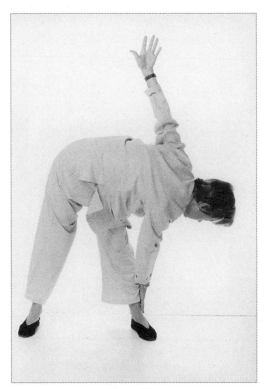

Photo 82

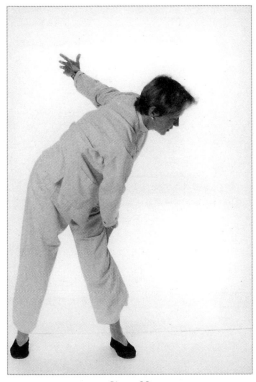

Photo 83

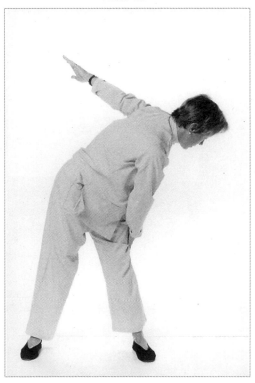

Photo 84

3
The Three Enemies:
Stress, Anxiety, and Emotionalism

Chinese medical practitioners were the first to introduce the concept of psychosomatic disturbances and have long studied the relationship between body and psyche, health and emotions. Strong emotions, whether negative or positive, are in the long run damaging to the health.

According to traditional Chinese doctors, every violent or prolonged emotion alters the energetic state of the organ it influences. For example, as even we in the West know, anger undermines the liver. Chinese medicine lists seven principal emotions to keep under control: joy, anger, fear, love, sorrow, hatred, and desire. Each of the five principal organs is associated with a particular emotion, which excess can transform into a pathological sentiment, thus upsetting the energetic circulation of the associated organ.

The organ/emotion/pathological emotion combinations are as follows:

- Liver / ardor / anger
- Heart / joy / overexcitement
- Spleen / worry / obsession
- Lungs / sadness / depression
- Kidneys / anxiety / fear
  (See Table 1 in Chapter 1 for the relationships of the five elements.)

If the energetic imbalance is prolonged, illness will arise—whether physical or mental depends on the individual case. Let us look at an example: If we consider the lungs, we see that in the table of the five elements this organ is associated with sadness. Sadness or grief that goes on a long time can cause confusion in the qi energy of the lungs. If this energy is depleted over a long period of time, the person becomes lymphatic and tires easily. Eventually, more serious illnesses will surface (asthma, chronic bronchitis, dermatological disturbances, a lowering of immune defenses, depression, and so forth). In the case of the heart, the most dangerous emotion is overexcitement—even too much joy, if it is violent. In fact, heart attacks are not uncommon in the "lucky" winners of the lottery.

It is therefore wise to keep a close eye on excessive emotions. Women have a propensity to be emotional, so we must control ourselves in this area. We must try not to become too agitated or worried, to give too much weight to things of no importance, or to wear ourselves out in exhausting discussions. The Taoist philosopher Lao-Tzu said that wisdom lies in the middle way. So seek as much as possible to preserve your peace and serenity. The practice of therapeutic sounds will help you to do this.

Therapeutic Sounds

Therapeutic sounds are another field in which the Chinese have been pioneers. More than two thousand years ago they discovered that certain sounds exerted a beneficial effect on our bodies, because their vibrations have the power to harmonize the energy of specific organs and regulate energetic circulation in their associated meridians. They also discovered that the utterance of these sounds had a calming effect on the nervous system and cerebral cortex. The only equivalent we have of this tradition in our Western culture is the Gregorian chant.

The sound can be a mantra (a sacred word or phrase), such as the famous Tibetan "Om," or it can follow a more technical system, whether Taoist or Buddhist, that brings sounds and organs into relationship with each other (Table 2).

In the Taoist system the sounds are whispered, whereas in the Buddhist system they are uttered with force and resonance. To practice the sounds, proceed as follows:

Stand or sit on a chair or on the ground with your legs crossed and your back straight. Cross your hands over the organ associated with the sound you are about to emit, covering your right hand with your left. Close your eyes and concentrate on the vibrations of the sound while seeking to direct it mentally toward the organ concerned. Inflate your abdomen as you inhale. When you exhale, contract your abdominal muscles while uttering the sound, so that it "comes out of the belly." Do not prolong the sound after you have finished exhaling; simply inhale again and repeat the exercise at least 20 times, using the same sound (see Photos 85 and 86).

Note: for "Shu" (pronounced *Sheeyu)* keep your eyes very widely opened; for "Chui" point the tip of your tongue toward the upper incisors, so as to complete an uninterrupted circle of energy between the median frontal meridian, Ren Mai, and the dorsal meridian, Du Mai. If you wish to work with a series of sounds during the course of the same exercise, pronounce each sound at least six times in a row, mentally directing its vibrations to the appropriate organ. The Chinese say that the more strongly and clearly the sound emerges, the more attuned is the energy of the organ. Try it! You will feel a noticeable sense of well-being right away.

Table 2: Therapeutic Sounds					
Corresponding Organ	Liver	Heart	Spleen	Lungs	Kidneys
The Taoist sounds	"Shu"	"Khe"	"Hu"	"Ssss"	"Chui"
The Buddhist sounds	"Pa"	"Haa"	"Mei"	"Ni"	"Hong"

The Three Enemies: Stress, Anxiety, and Emotionalism

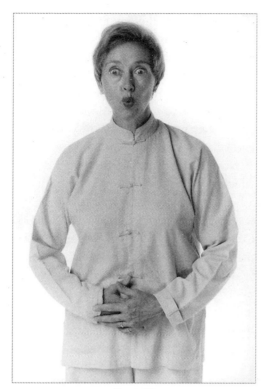

Photo 85

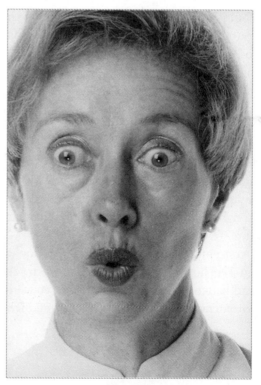

Photo 86

Dantian Breathing: Visualization of the Pink Balloon

"The pink balloon" is an autogenic training exercise that combines body, mind, breathing, and visualization. Aside from inducing calm and complete relaxation, it stimulates all the internal organs, thanks to abdominal respiration. It is therefore particularly helpful in regulating intestinal functions; resolving abdominal problems such as gas, indigestion, and gastritis; and curing insomnia.

There are two ways to engage in this exercise. You can learn it by heart and then practice it with full recall of all its details or you can let yourself be guided by someone else who reads it to you step by step. In the latter case, whoever is guiding you should speak very slowly and softly, maintaining an even tone so as to establish a climate conducive to relaxation. A goal of this exercise is for the practitioner to reach an alpha state, combining perfect relaxation with acuity and awareness of mind.

You will be visualizing the energies that circulate throughout your body and the color pink of the air filling your abdomen as you feel a calming effect on both body and psyche. Remember: abdominal breathing; the color pink; and the therapeutic sound "Ssss," hissed through the teeth.

You can do this exercise standing up, seated, or lying down. Lying down is preferable, as it favors total relaxation. Stretch out on your back on the ground or floor with your legs straight, your heels touching each other, and your chin slightly pulled in. Place your left hand on your breast over the heart and your right hand below your navel on the dantian (see Figure 9).

First concentrate your attention on your lower abdomen. Feel how your stomach inflates when you inhale and flattens when you exhale. Then concentrate your attention on your chest: You should feel no movement at all in your rib cage under the palm of your right hand. You should be able to feel instead the beating of your heart. Focus for a moment on the regular rhythm of this beating; listen to your heart. Then remove your hand from your chest and bring it down to cover your other hand, resting low on the stomach. Feel again how your abdomen rises and falls (see Photos 87 and 88).

Now imagine that you are inhaling soft pink air, which is little by little filling up your belly. Think of a balloon: When you inhale, the pink balloon inflates; when you exhale, the pink balloon deflates. Continue like this for several minutes, visualizing the color pink—so soft, so sweet, so calming.

After a while begin to affirm these words in your mind: "relax," as you inhale and the pink balloon inflates; and "subside," as you exhale and the pink balloon deflates. Repeat these inner affirmations until they integrate perfectly with your breathing. At this point modify the second affirmation by replacing it with the sound "Ssss," hissed audibly while you exhale. Continue in this manner until the sound becomes fainter and fainter, then almost inaudible, and until your body is completely relaxed, in a perfect state of calm.

To conclude the exercise, bring your awareness back into your mind, move your hands and feet, stretch yourself in every direction, sit up, and massage your face and head with the tips of your fingers. Finally, cross your hands with the left over the right on your lower stomach and bring the energy back to the dantian.

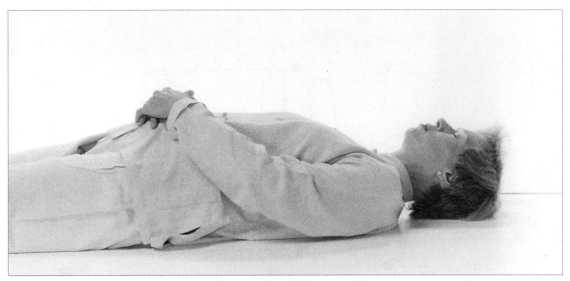

Photo 87

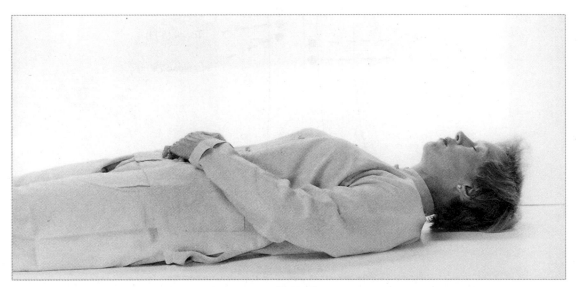

Photo 88

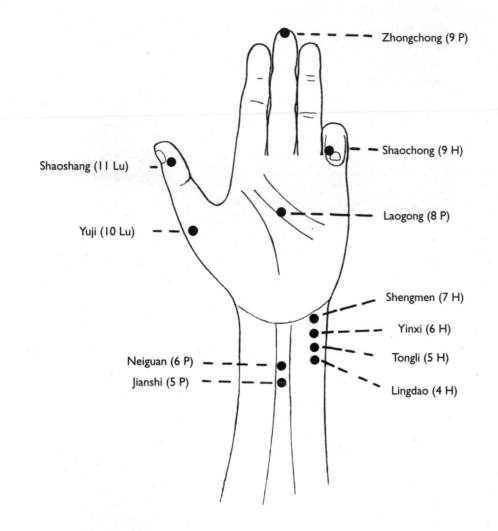

Shaoshang (11 Lu)

Yuji (10 Lu)

Zhongchong (9 P)

Shaochong (9 H)

Laogong (8 P)

Shengmen (7 H)

Yinxi (6 H)

Neiguan (6 P)

Jianshi (5 P)

Tongli (5 H)

Lingdao (4 H)

Figure 11: The antistress points of the hand and wrist

The Three Enemies: Stress, Anxiety, and Emotionalism

Acupressure on Antistress Points

To calm "the fire of the heart" to assuage anger, anxiety, and nervousness, it is useful to employ a few digital acupressure exercises that can be performed even in situations of stress. The points involved belong mostly to the meridians of the organs most influenced by anxiety: the heart, the pericardium, and the liver. To locate the points, study Figures 11 to 13.

Exert pressure for several minutes on the points listed below. Start in every case by inhaling, then press while you exhale.

- *Neiguan* (6 P), about 2 "distances," or cun (see Figure 3 for an explanation of the measurements), above the fold on the inside of the wrist between the two flexor tendons

- *Lingdao* (4 H), 1½ cun above the fold on the inside of the wrist to the outside of the anterior cubital tendon
- *Tongli* (5 H), beneath *Lingdao,* 1 cun above the fold on the inside of the wrist
- *Yinxi* (6 H), next under *Tongli,* ½ cun above the fold on the inside of the wrist
- *Shengmen* (7 H), beneath *Yinxi,* exactly on the fold on the inside of the wrist
- *Taichong* (3 Lv), in the space between the first and second toes, 1½ cun above their juncture
- *Ququan* (8 Lv), at the inside edge of the crease in the back of the knee

Also massage up and down the whole area of the sternum.

This therapy can be concluded with a massage of the meridians of the arms (see Chapter 4).

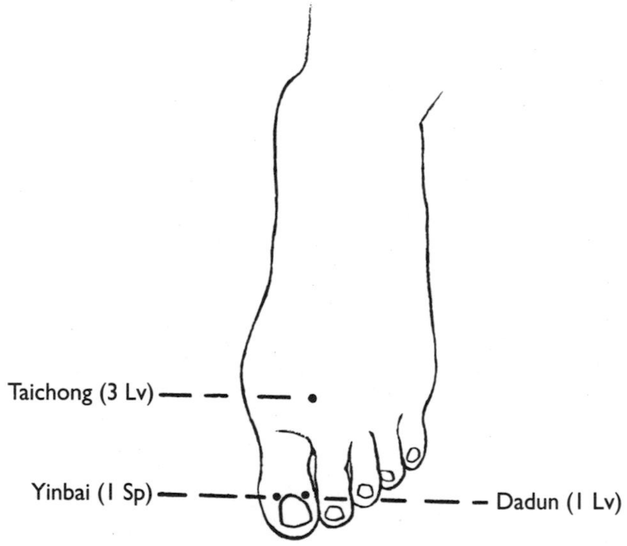

Taichong (3 Lv) — — —

Yinbai (1 Sp) — — — — — Dadun (1 Lv)

Figure 12: The antistress points of the top of the foot

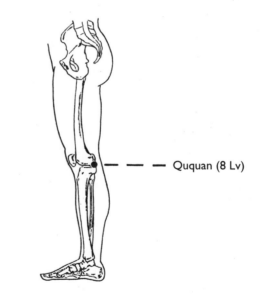

— — — Ququan (8 Lv)

Figure 13: The antistress point of the knee

4
How to Stay in Great Shape

Massaging the Meridians

(five minutes)

Massaging the inside and outside of your arms and legs can in just a few minutes give your whole body an energetic charge, since it stimulates at least 12 acupuncture points.

This exercise is very useful for people who stay seated for long hours, because it combats stagnation of the blood in the legs and therefore prevents cramps and varicose veins. It also helps to combat high blood pressure, water retention throughout the body, and excess weight.

You can do this exercise standing up or sitting down. Massage each limb 12 times in a row every morning—every evening too if you have circulatory problems. Inhale when the direction of the massage is toward the trunk; exhale when the direction of the massage is toward the extremities. *Be sure to massage in the indicated direction.*

Massaging the Arms. Place your right hand on your chest near the left shoulder, then slide your palm in a continuous motion down the inside of your left arm, ending at the fingertips of your left palm. Turn your left arm over and slide your right palm up the outside of the arm until you reach the shoulder. Lightly press the point *Jianjing* (21 GB), in the small hollow above the shoulder blade (see Figure 8). Repeat 11 more times. Then perform the same massage using your left hand on your right arm (see Photos 89 to 100).

Massaging the Legs. Sit down, on the floor if possible. Starting from the inner edge of the feet, massage upward along the inside of your legs and thighs until you reach the groin. Then slide your hands down over your hips and down the outside of your legs. Keep your thumbs and the palms of your hands widely separated, so that you can simultaneously massage the sides and backs of your legs (see Photos 101 to 112).

Once you have learned this exercise, start mentally following the flow of energy ascending and descending along the meridians.

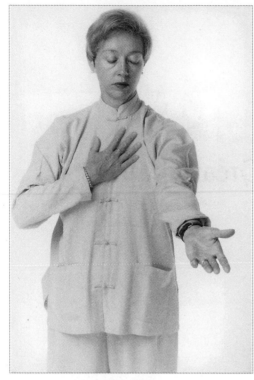

Photo 89

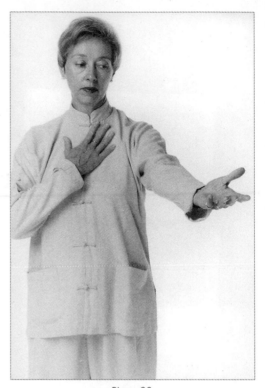

Photo 90

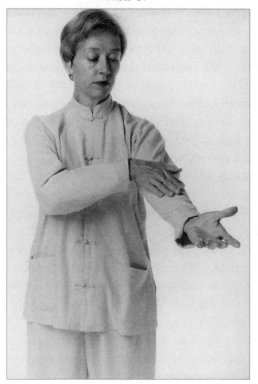

Photo 91

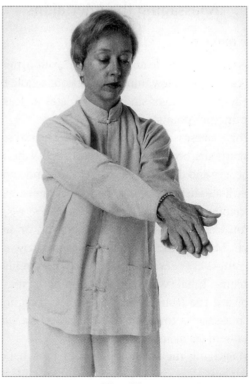

Photo 92

How to Stay in Great Shape

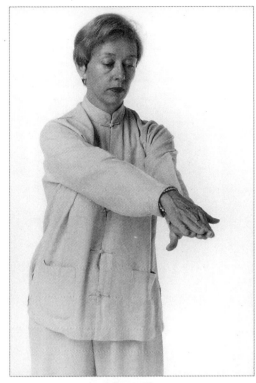

Photo 93

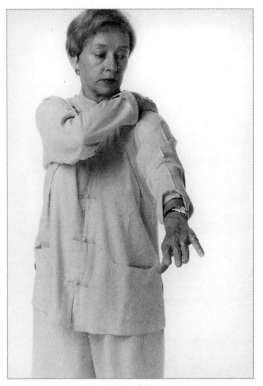

Photo 94

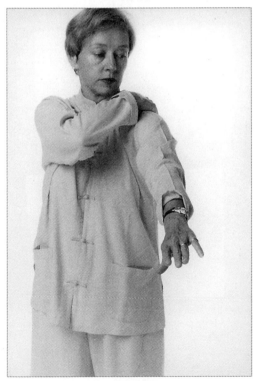

Photo 95

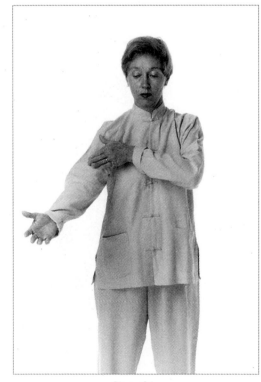

Photo 96

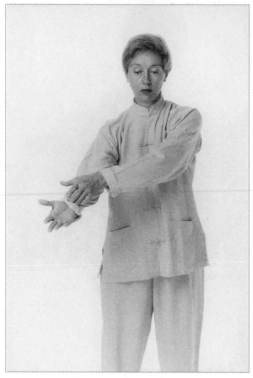

Photo 97

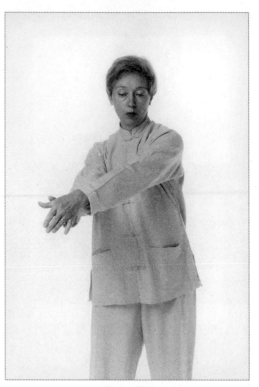

Photo 98

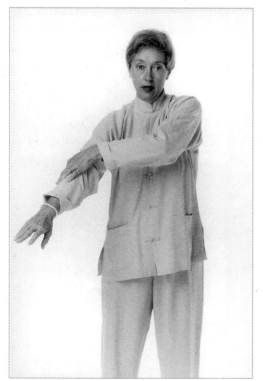

Photo 99

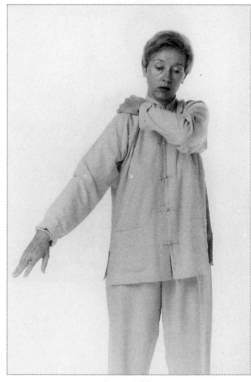

Photo 100

How to Stay in Great Shape

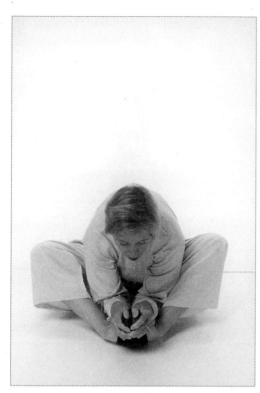

Photo 101

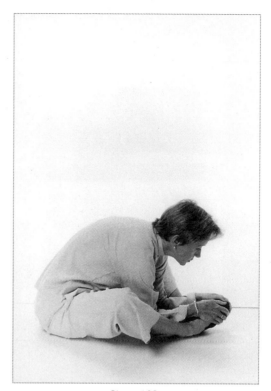

Photo 102

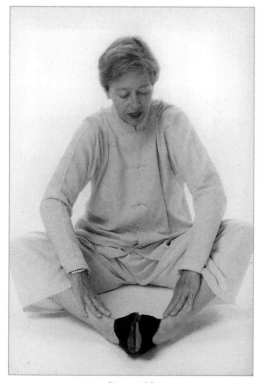

Photo 103

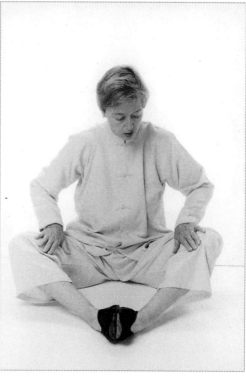

Photo 104

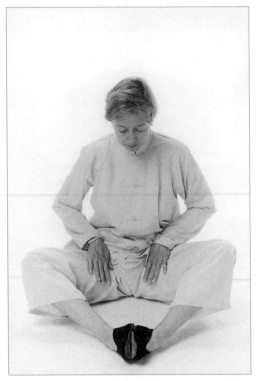

Photo 105

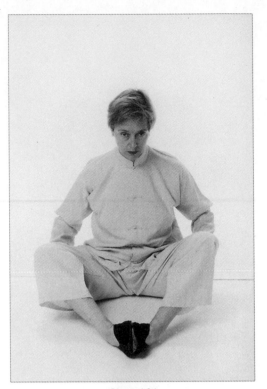

Photo 106

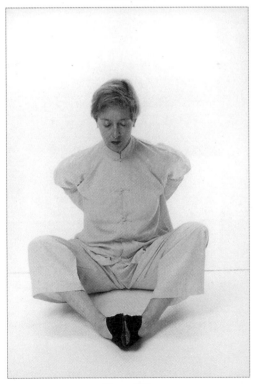

Photo 107

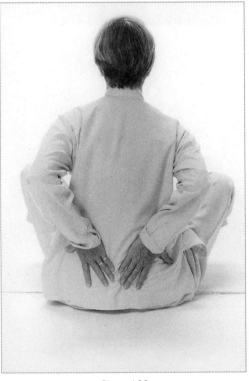

Photo 108

How to Stay in Great Shape

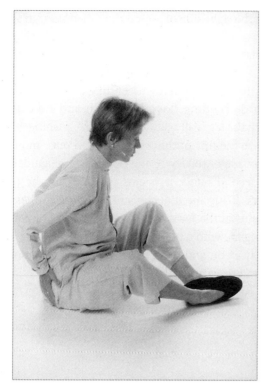

Photo 109

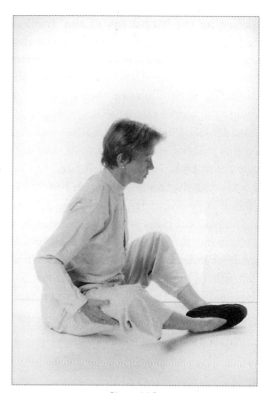

Photo 110

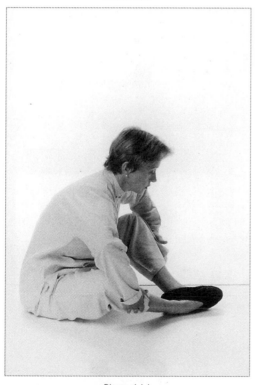

Photo 111

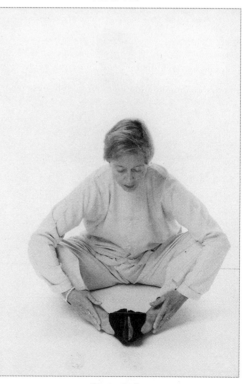

Photo 112

Massaging the Meridians of the Trunk. Performed in the morning, this quick exercise (two to three minutes) circulates energy in the whole upper part of the body. It alleviates tiredness in the shoulders and if done rapidly warms you up in a hurry. It stimulates the meridians of the lungs, kidneys, and gall bladder (see Photos 113 to 120).

Do this exercise standing up with your legs set slightly apart. Hold your open left hand in front of your body with the thumb resting on your pubis. As you inhale, move your left hand upward along the median line of the body until it reaches the level of the collarbone; then open your palm on your chest and slide it under your left armpit and down along the left side of the body while you exhale, until it reaches midthigh. Then place your right hand on your pubis and slide it in the exact same motion over the right side of your torso. Then start up again with your left hand; in other words, alternate hands, so that as one is climbing, the other is descending.

Once you have learned the exercise, mentally follow the flow of energy ascending along the trunk, then descending down the thigh and from there down the leg (gall bladder meridian), rushing all the way to the tips of the toes to ascend once more up the inside of the leg to the pubis, where, guided by the second hand, it begins to climb up the torso again. "This mental concentration multiplies the benefits of the massage," insists Doctor Grace Yu of Shanghai, who taught me the exercise. "With a little practice you will soon feel a beneficial sensation of warmth in your limbs."

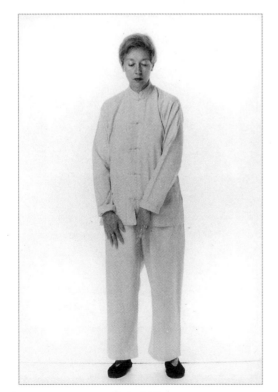

Photo 113

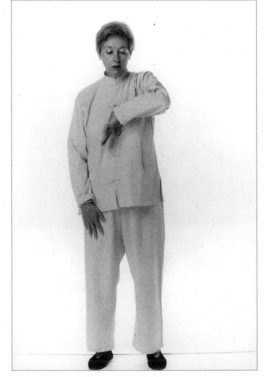

Photo 114

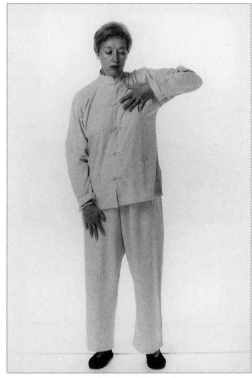

Photo 115

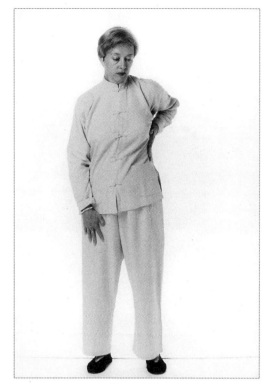

Photo 116

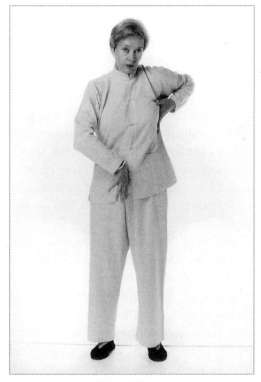

Photo 117

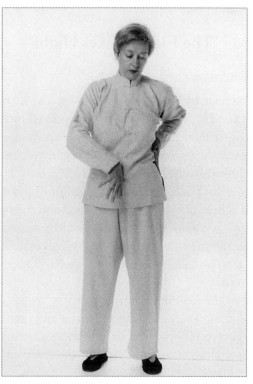

Photo 118

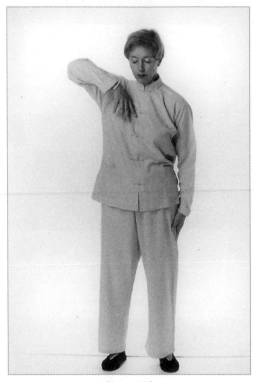

Photo 119

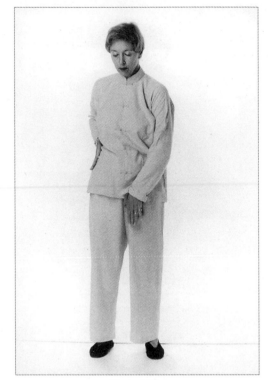

Photo 120

"The Hawk Takes Flight"

(five minutes)

Exercise by Mas Rodgers. This exercise strengthens the sight (which is why it is associated with the hawk), relaxes the shoulders, and improves energetic circulation in the meridian of the liver, the organ linked to the eyes and the sound "Xu." It also relaxes the brain by bringing blood to it when the head is held in a downward position and stimulates the *Shu* points of the bladder meridian located between the shoulder blades. The last part of the exercise relaxes the lumbar region, often a repository for tensions.

If at the beginning you are unable to roll your hands completely over, cross them behind your back and persevere—you will do it sooner or later!

Contraindication: Skip Part 5 of this exercise if you suffer from high blood pressure—no exceptions!

Start by standing very straight with your feet slightly apart and holding your hands behind your back with fingers laced together and palms facing up (see Photo 121).

1. (see Photo 122): While inhaling, keeping your fingers laced together, turn your palms to the outside and continue turning them until they face the ground. At the same time, raise your shoulders slightly, bend your back so that it curves gently outward, and look up. At the end of your inhalation, push your palms downward. Pause for a moment in this position.

2. (see Photos 123 and 124): As you inhale, let your shoulders drop while your hands rotate in the opposite direction, toward your body and then downward, until the palms face down once again. Your arms should be fully outstretched and your shoulder blades pushed close together. Concentrate on the *Shu* points of the bladder meridian located between the shoulder blades (see Figure 8), as these points are stimulated during this phase of the exercise.

How to Stay in Great Shape

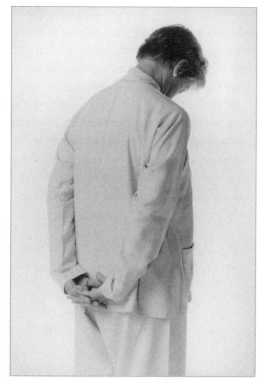

Photo 121

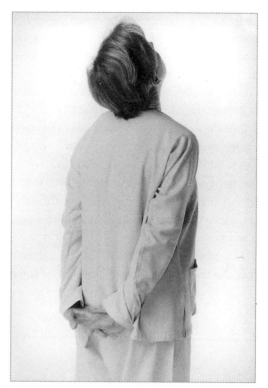

Photo 122

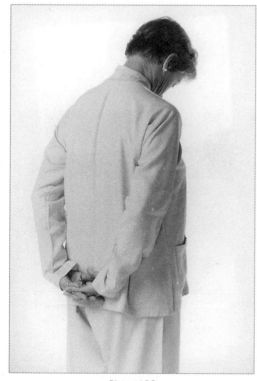

Photo 123

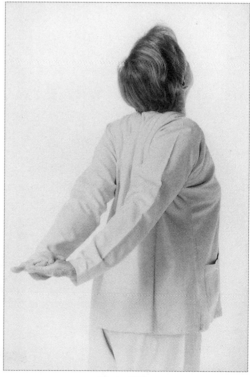

Photo 124

Accompany the movement by lowering your head onto your chest. Avoid any arch to the spine by tilting the bottom of your pelvis forward. Pause, then inhale again while rotating your palms in the opposite direction until they regain their original position. Repeat the exercise three times.

3. (see Photo 125): After your last exhalation, inhale and lean forward, bending your body only at the waist with your back straight and your chin out. At the same time, lift your arms behind your back with your fingers laced together; raise them as high as you can without straining. Pause in this position for a moment.

4. (see Photos 126 to 128): As you exhale, pronounce the therapeutic sound "Xuuu . . . ," lowering your hands, separating them, and placing the palms on your lower back on either side of your spine, then sliding them down the backs of your thighs and legs to your heels and along the outside of the feet, over the toes until you touch the big toe.

5. (see Photo 129): At the end of your exhalation, keep this position, letting your head and arms droop naturally and relaxing your body completely while you look between your legs and behind you. In this position take in a few half breaths, followed by complete exhalations accompanied by the sound "Xuuu . . . ."

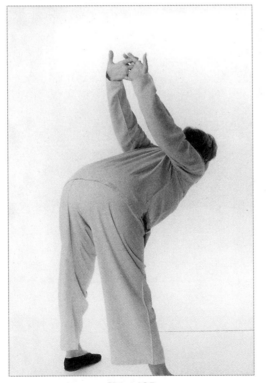

Photo 125

How to Stay in Great Shape

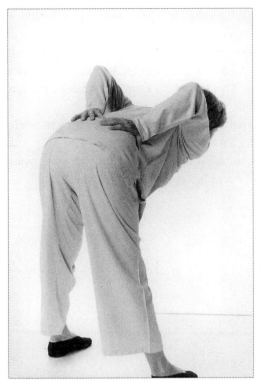

Photo 126

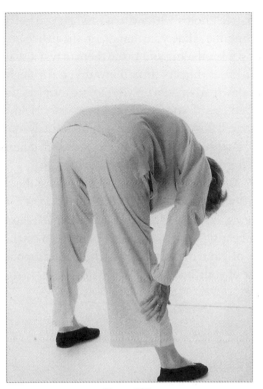

Photo 127

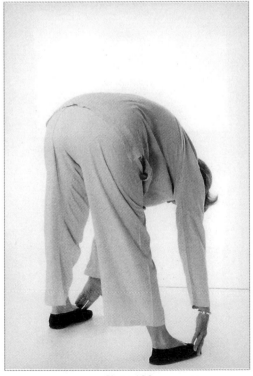

Photo 128

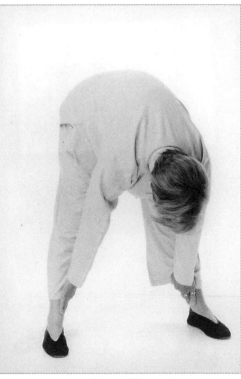

Photo 129

6. (see Photos 130 and 131): When you feel ready to continue, slide your hands up the inside of your legs while inhaling and bring them to rest just above your knees, fingers turned inward on the thighs, as you slowly straighten up your torso. Your legs should be bent, as if you were on horseback. Hold your torso well forward and your spine absolutely straight: This is a position that stretches the lumbar muscles and is greatly to their benefit.

7. (see Photos 132 to 138): Keeping the same position, turn your head to the left and exhale while uttering the sound "Xuuu . . ." over the left shoulder and bearing down with your right hand on the inside of your right thigh, which is now supporting most of your body weight. Do not strain.

Turn your head to the front again and inhale. Then turn your head to the right and exhale while uttering the sound "Xuuu . . ." over the right shoulder, bearing down with your left hand on your inner left thigh. This part of the exercise unblocks the lumbar region.

Finally, inhale again, facing front; then while exhaling slowly straighten yourself up, pronouncing the sound "Xuuu . . . ." Finish by crossing your left hand over your right on the dantian.

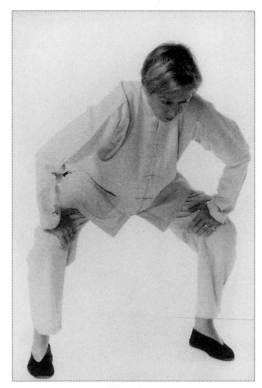

Photo 130

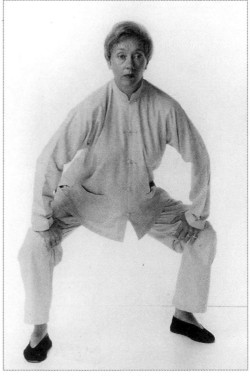

Photo 131

How to Stay in Great Shape

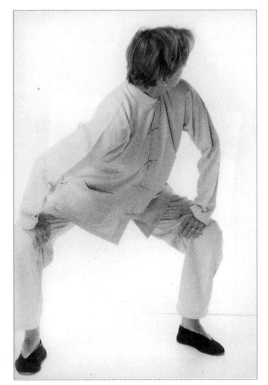

Photo 132

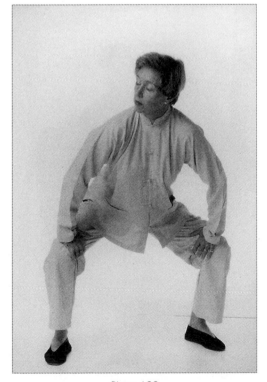

Photo 133

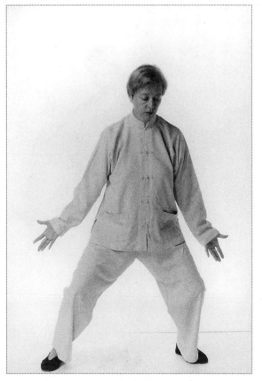

Photo 134

How to Stay in Great Shape

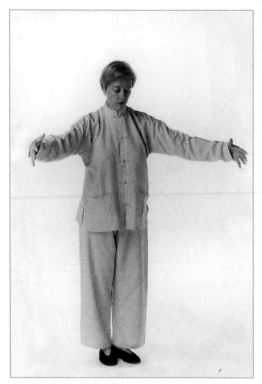

Photo 135

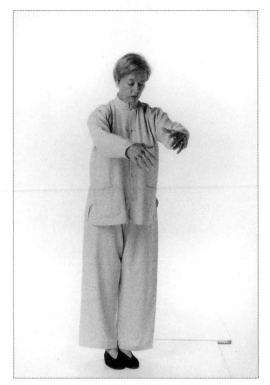

Photo 136

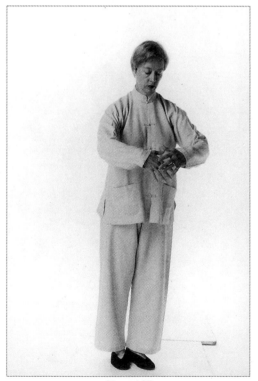

Photo 137

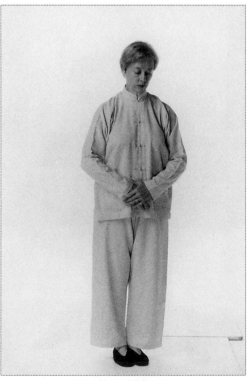

Photo 138

How to Stay in Great Shape

"Greeting to the Sky and Earth"

(three minutes)

Exercise by Mas Rodgers. This exercise stretches and tones the vertebral column (see Photos 139 to 146). The therapeutic sound used is "Hiiii . . . ," the *H* fully aspirated, the *i* sounding like "eeee." This sound is linked to the meridian of the pericardium (P), as well as the meridian of the three cavities, or triple heater (TH)—the thorax and upper and lower abdomen. This last meridian regulates the thyroid and the metabolism.

Stand straight, set your legs straight, your arms to your sides. As you inhale, place your hands on the front of your thighs and slide them up your body, just barely brushing it, until they reach your chest. Then,

raising your elbows, slide your hands upward along the ears and raise them over your head, stretching your arms fully. Your palms should be facing each other with your fingertips pointing toward the sky. During the inhalation, mentally follow the flow of qi coming up through your feet from the earth and rising through the movements of your hands up into your brain.

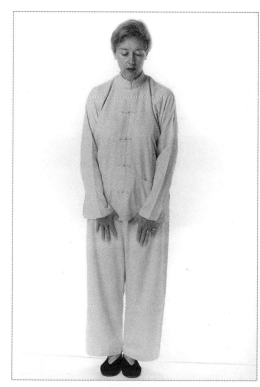

Photo 139

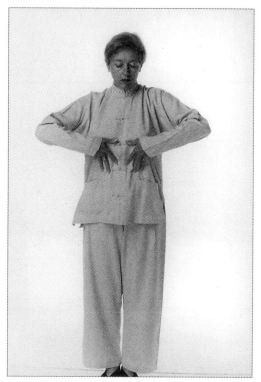

Photo 140

While you exhale, take one step to the right so that your feet are in line with your hips, turn your palms so that they face frontward, then lean forward, bending only your waist, without arching your back or bending your knees, and push into the air in front of you with your hands and arms outstretched and your wrists bent back, until your torso and arms are parallel to the ground. Then bend your back as well and lean down until you touch your toes, with your arms relaxed. During the whole exhalation, pronounce the sound "Hiiii . . ." softly, drawing it out for as long as possible.

While inhaling, slowly straighten your body, vertebra after vertebra, visualizing the progressive straightening of the lumbar, then the dorsal, then the cervical vertebrae as your hands slide up the inside of your legs and thighs and then along the front part of your torso, as in the first inhalation of the exercise.

Repeat the exercise until you feel that your spine is completely relaxed.

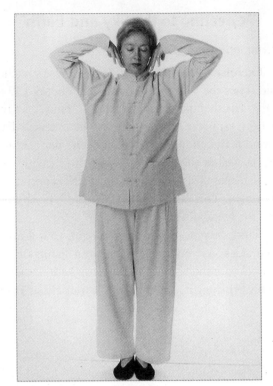

Photo 141

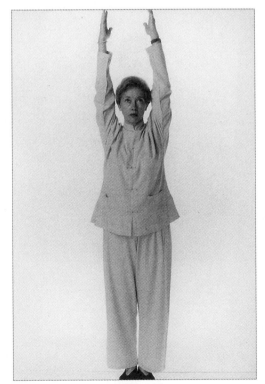

Photo 142

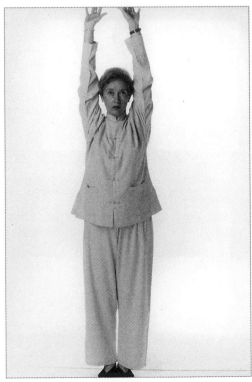

Photo 143

How to Stay in Great Shape

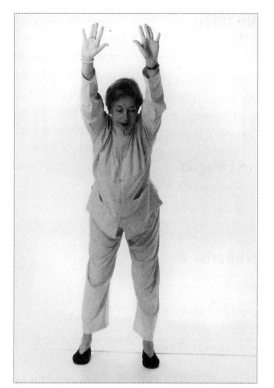

Photo 144

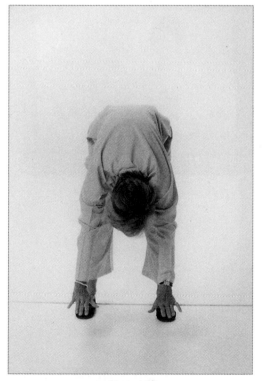

Photo 145

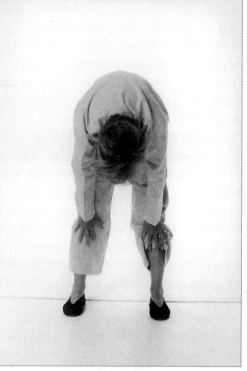

Photo 146

Stimulating the Mingmen, the Door of Life

(three minutes)

Mingmen (4 DM), the "Door of Life," is the receptacle for the special energy of the kidneys. For its position on the spine and the way to stimulate it, see Figure 8 and the accompanying text in Chapter 1.

The Six Circles of the Dragon

(eight minutes)

This exercise is described in full in the second section of Chapter 2.

Opening the Meridians

(three to five minutes per meridian)

Exercise Taught by the European Institute of Qigong. When performing these exercises, start on the side of the body that is loosest. Repeat three to eight times on both sides.

Stomach Meridian

The human body, connected to the entire universe, is sensitive to external disturbances. When the meridian of the stomach is disturbed in a serious way, the following pathologies may manifest themselves: tooth decay; pains in the jaw, collarbone, legs, and knee-caps; tendinitis; muscular contractions such as cramps; and a feeling of oppression in the chest. These pathologies can be accompanied by stomach pains or aches. To remedy the situation, you must open and "iron" the meridian of the stomach in such a way as to unblock and energize it (see Photos 147 to 154).

Take a step forward with your left foot, resting it on the heel only so that the sole remains in the air, and inhale with your hands crossed over your breast. Then exhale, resting your body weight on your bent right leg, while your hands slide down the front of your outstretched left leg all the way to the toes, "ironing" the left foot so that the sole is now flat on the ground. Meanwhile, shift your body weight onto your left leg. Now curl the toes of your right foot, which is still behind you, and lift up your sole and heel so that the foot is resting on the second toe, the termination point of the meridian of the stomach. Inhale again, and bring your arms and clasped hands to describe an arc from the left foot to complete extension above the head. Pause in this position for a moment, then exhale while bringing your hands down and crossing them on your chest. Inhale and perform the same sequence of movements on the right side. Follow the movements of your hands with your glance.

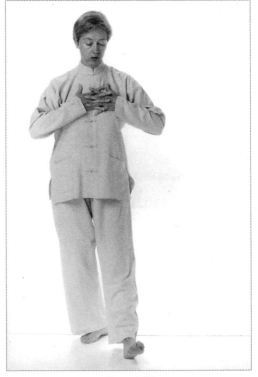

Photo 147

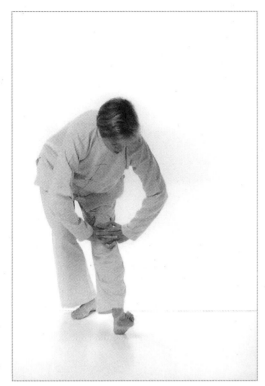

Photo 148

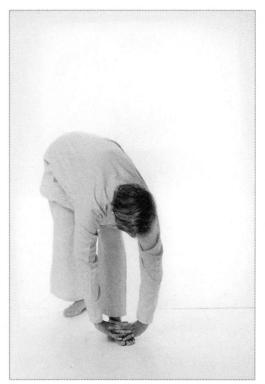

Photo 149

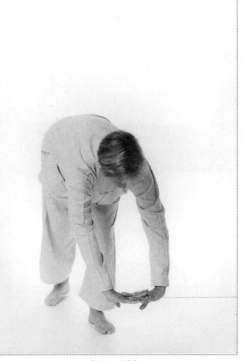

Photo 150

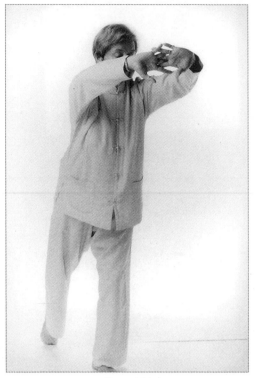

Photo 151

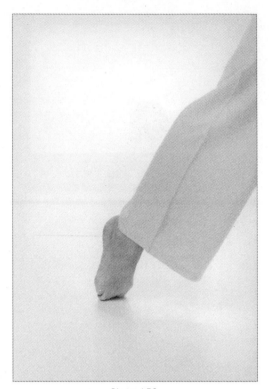

Photo 152

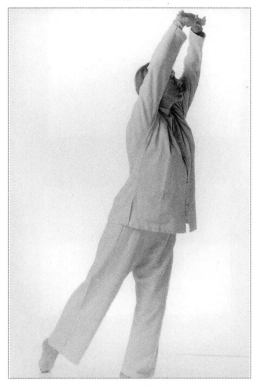

Photo 153

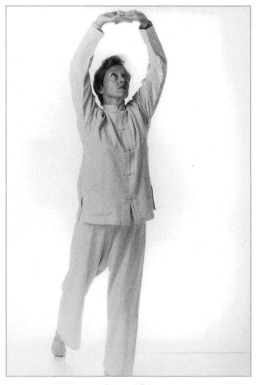

Photo 154

How to Stay in Great Shape

Spleen Meridian

Hold your legs as wide apart as possible, feet and knees open, torso erect, hands on your hips. Inhale; then, while you are exhaling, bend your right knee, turning your torso and head toward your fully out-stretched left leg. Meanwhile, turn the front of your left foot toward the inside, lifting the big toe up from the ground. Perform the same movements to the right while flexing your left knee (see Photos 155 to 157).

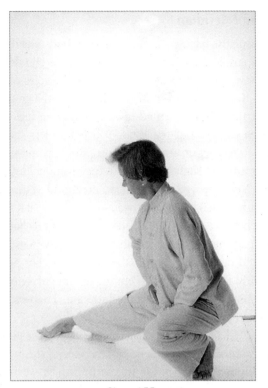

Photo 155

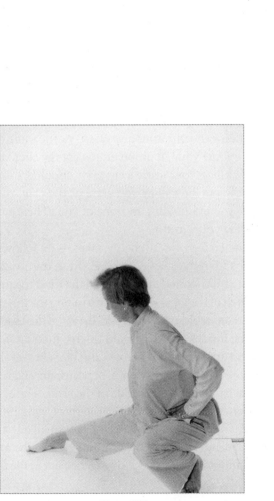

Photo 156

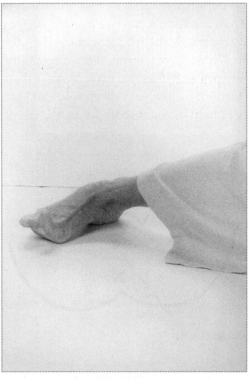

Photo 157

Lung Meridian

Assume the basic position of qigong: body erect, feet set apart so that they are in line with the shoulders, body weight distributed evenly over the soles of the feet. Keep your toes in firm contact with the ground, their tips slightly turned inward, and your legs and knees straight but not rigid. Your shoulders should be relaxed, your arms held naturally to your sides, your armpits slightly open as if they were holding an egg. Keep your back and head erect and your chin slightly pulled back. Your head should feel as if it were attached to a string that connects the point *Baihui* (20 DM), at the top of the cranium, to the sky. Your face should be relaxed. Thrust the bottom of your pelvis slightly forward, so as to eliminate any curvature of the spine and render it flat and straight. This position strengthens the muscles of the buttocks.

Visualize an upsidedown Y connecting the points *Yongquan* (1 K, at the center of the sole of the foot—see Figure 5), *Huiyin* (on the perinium, between the vagina and the anus—see Figure 14), and *Baihui* (20 DM, at the top of the head). Cross your hands under your navel on the dantian (see Photo 158), the right hand covered by the left for women, the left hand covered by the right for men, superimposing the two *Laogong* points (8 P) located in the center of the palms (see Figure 6). Close your eyes halfway and gaze directly in front of you without focusing.

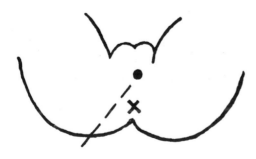

Huiyin (1 RM)

Figure 14: The Huiyin point

Photos 158 to 165 illustrate this exercise. Close your eyes and rest the tip of your tongue on the arch of the palate. Slowly swallow your saliva, mentally following its course down into the stomach.

Now inhale, while contracting your abdominal muscles and slowly lifting your relaxed arms (elbows slightly bent, palms facing the ground) to either side of your body without raising them above your shoulders.

As you exhale, slowly turn the palms of your hands outward to the front, concentrating on the movement of your thumbs, which are rotating backward and carrying the hands and forearms to a point a little behind the shoulders. This movement charges up the meridian of the lungs, which begins under the collarbone and ends in the thumb. Pause for a moment in this position, concentrating on the charge you can feel moving from your thumbs to your collarbone. Repeat these movements a number of times.

Now inhale, closing your two arms in a circle in front of your chest, one hand held over the other with fingers spread, as if you were squeezing a big ball between your arms and chest. At the same time concentrate your attention on the energy circulating down along your arms from your shoulders to the tips of your fingers as you stare at the "ball of energy" you are holding in front of you. Then pause, holding your breath.

The course the qi energy takes is as follows: It climbs from the soles of the feet (from the *Yongquan* point (1 K), located at the level of the third toe under the arch of the foot—see Figure 5) along the three yin meridians (spleen, liver, and kidneys) of the foot and up the insides of the legs and thighs. It continues to ascend up the front of the torso and branches off along the three yin meridians (lungs, pericardium, and heart) of the hand, down the inside of the arms. The qi also descends along the course of the three yang meridians (large intestine, triple heater, and small intestine) of the hand, along the outside and back of the arms. It continues its descent following the path of the three

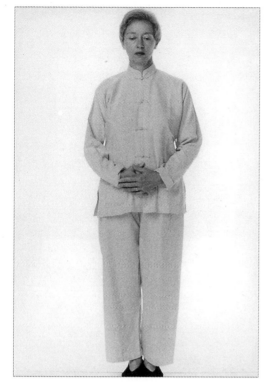

Photo 158

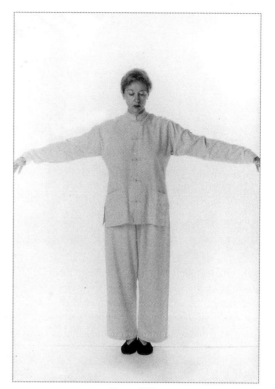

Photo 159

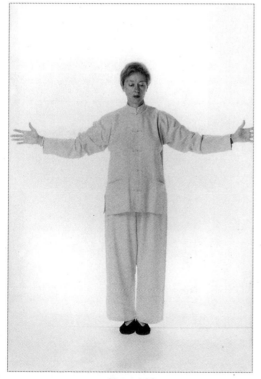

Photo 160

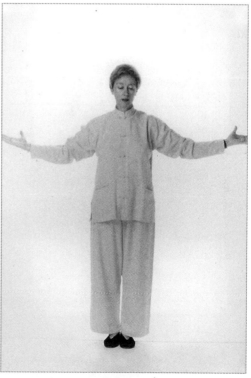

Photo 161

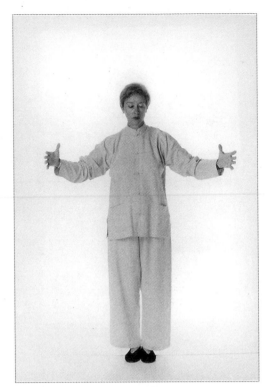

Photo 162

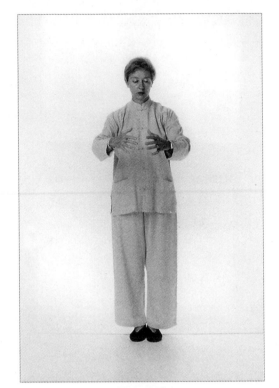

Photo 163

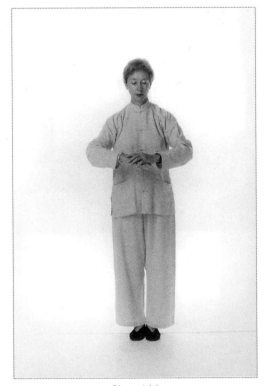

Photo 164

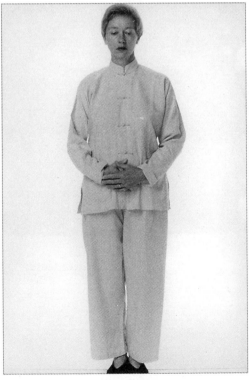

Photo 165

How to Stay in Great Shape

yang meridians (stomach, gall bladder, and bladder) of the foot, down the front, side, and back of the thighs, legs, and feet, respectively.

As you exhale, relax the tension in your abdomen, turn the palms of your hands toward the ground, and slowly push the sphere of energy downward. Then bring your hands toward your body and cross them once more on the dantian.

Large Intestine Meridian

This exercise begins with the opening of the meridian of the waist, the special *daimai* meridian (see Photos 166 to 174). Raise your arms horizontally in front of you up to the height of the shoulders with your palms facing down. As you then lower the arms, turn your palms up, place the edge of your hands on your waist, and follow the waist meridian around toward your hips in the back.

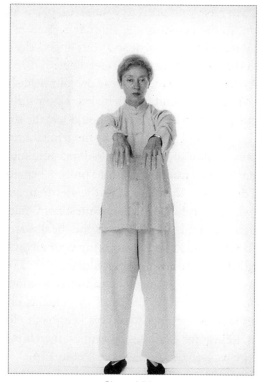

Photo 166

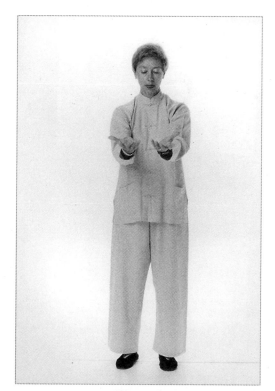

Photo 167

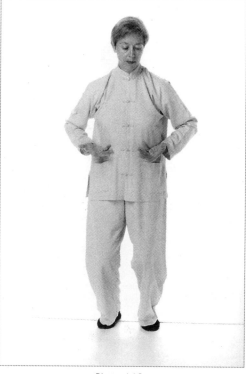

Photo 168

Then raise your arms to your sides, palms facing down, to the height of the shoulders. Your elbows and wrists should be bent and your fingers closed to form the "beak of the crane" (see Photo 170).

As you inhale, lean your head on your right shoulder while you extend your left arm (elbow still bent slightly, wrist still bent); you should feel the stretch in your arm and shoulder. This movement brings a certain tension to the sternocleidomastoid muscle, which extends from the mastoid process behind the ear, down past the clavical to the sternum, and to the whole meridian of the large intestine. While you stretch this muscle, be sure that the "beaks" are facing behind you as you try to bring your elbows forward without raising your shoulders.

As you exhale, return to your initial position and perform the same sequence of movements on the other side. Remember to always keep your elbows bent. Repeat the exercise eight times, then bring the energy back to the dantian (see Photo 174).

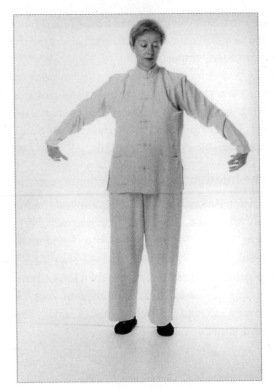

Photo 169

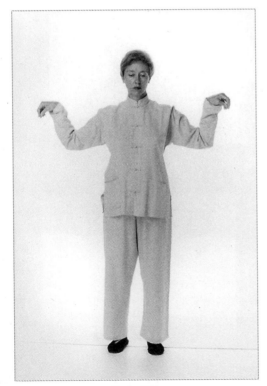

Photo 170

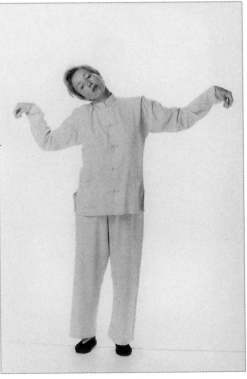

Photo 171

How to Stay in Great Shape

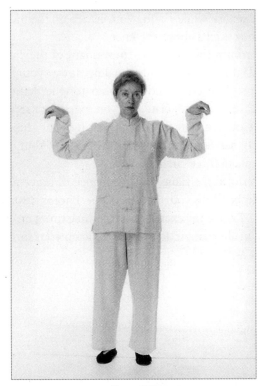

Photo 172

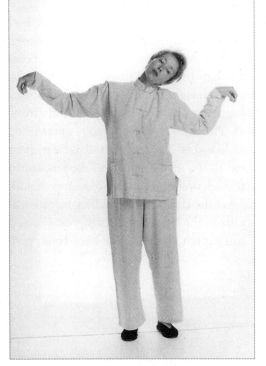

Photo 173

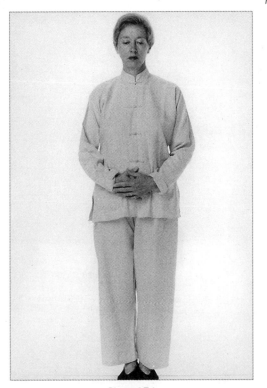

Photo 174

Kidney Meridian

Spread your legs as widely as you can and, holding your torso perfectly straight, go down in a knee bend on your right knee until you are sitting (if possible) on your right heel (see Photos 175 to 179). Meanwhile, the left leg remains straight and outstretched, with the front of the foot raised slightly from the ground. Place your hands, fingers spread, on the ground like this: The right hand is near the right foot and to the inside of it, and the left hand near the left thigh and to the inside of it. You should distinctly feel the course of the kidney meridian along the inside of the left leg and thigh.

If you cannot complete the knee bend, perform the exercise while resting your hands on the insides of your thighs above the knee.

Perform the following "movement of the crane's head" three times: While inhaling, lower your chin against your chest and curl your tongue, letting it touch the upper palate. As you exhale, raise your head and elongate your neck, jutting your chin forward; then let it drop to your chest again. Your head will make three circles.

Perform the same exact sequence of movements while bending your left knee (see Photos 180 and 181). Repeat the exercise at least three times on each side in alternation. Remember to keep your torso as erect as possible.

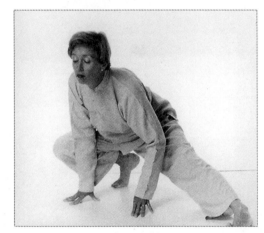

Photo 175

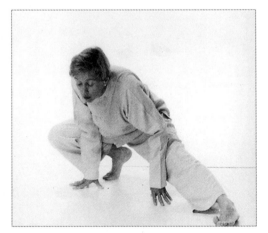

Photo 176

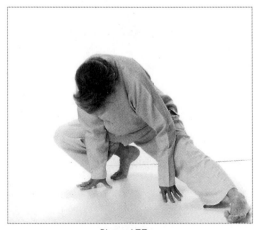

Photo 177

How to Stay in Great Shape

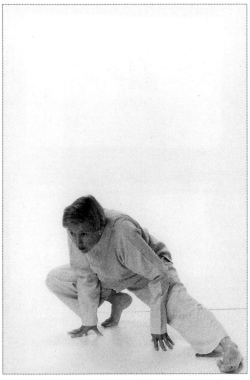

Photo 178

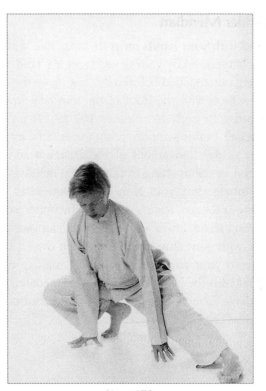

Photo 179

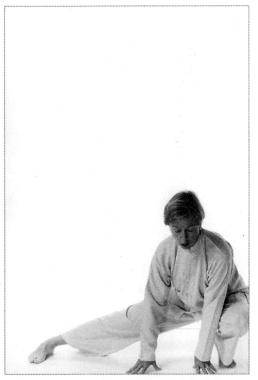

Photo 180

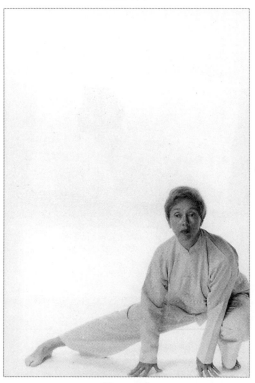

Photo 181

Bladder Meridian

Stand with your hands on your hips, your straight torso supported by your flexed right leg; hold your left leg outstretched before you, resting on the heel of the foot, with the front of the foot bent inward toward your body (see Photos 182 to 191 for this exercise). In this position, begin the exercise by performing the "movement of the crane's head" described in the opening of the kidney meridian. As you inhale, drop your chin against your chest and curl your tongue, resting it against the upper palate. As you exhale, lower your head and elongate your neck with your chin jutting out, then drop it once more to your chest. Repeat twice, making three circles with the head, one small, one medium, and one large. The movement starts from the waist and involves the entire torso.

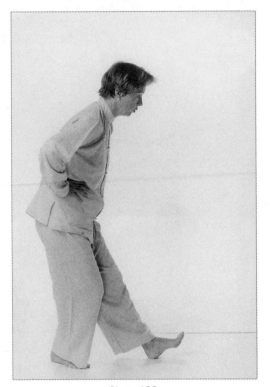

Photo 182

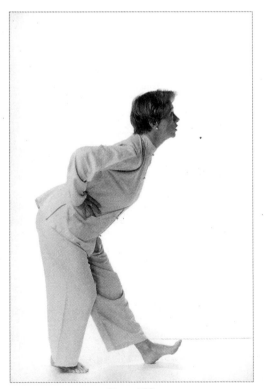

Photo 183

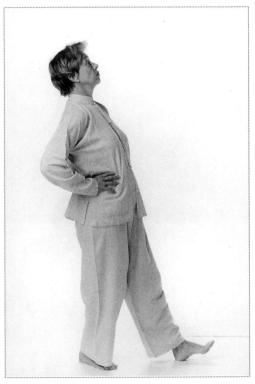

Photo 184

How to Stay in Great Shape

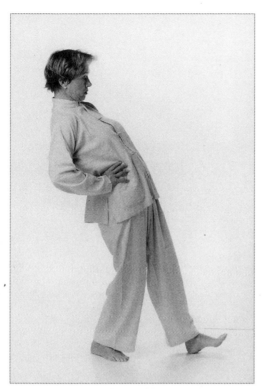

Photo 185

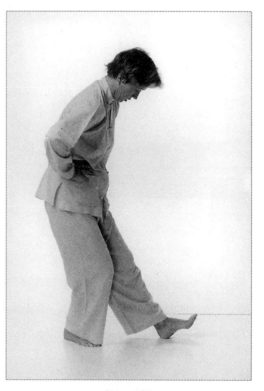

Photo 186

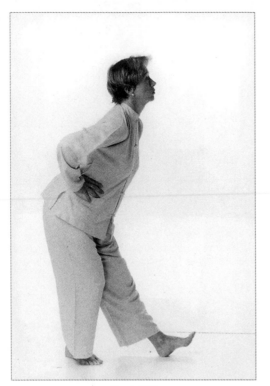

Photo 187

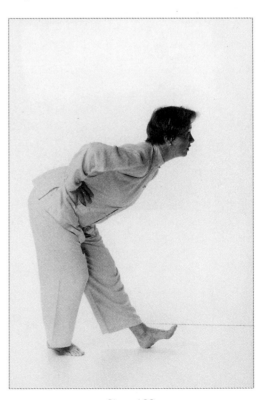

Photo 188

How to Stay in Great Shape

When you have completed the three circles, inhale again, pulling your chin in; then exhale while folding your torso forward onto your outstretched left leg and lowering your bent arms to the sides of the same leg. The front of your upper body should be almost resting on your left knee and your right leg is bent as deeply as possible. In this position you should feel the course of the bladder meridian down the front of the leg, in the back, and along the spine right up to the top of the head.

Perform the same movement on the other leg and repeat the exercise three times in alternation for each side.

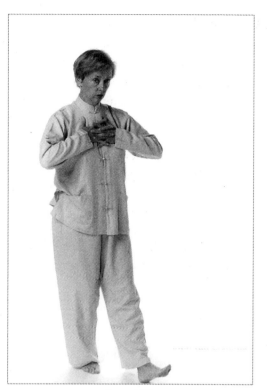

Photo 189

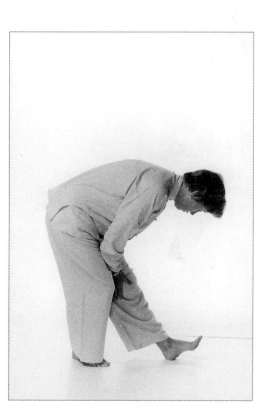

Photo 190

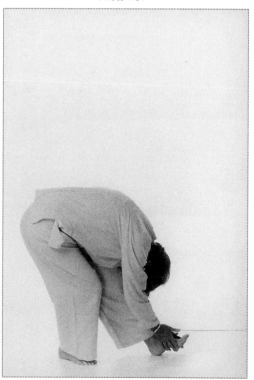

Photo 191

Liver Meridian

In cases of energy blockage along the liver meridian, the following disturbances may manifest: tendinitis, joint pains in the knees, muscular adynamia, or disturbances of the external genitals (premature or delayed ejaculation, "emotional" erection). If the energy is blocked for a long time, disturbances of memory may arise (the liver participates in this function), as well as disturbances of the digestive system and the venous system (varicose veins, cramps, hemorrhoids, or painful menstruation). Aside from these, a liver in bad condition often leads to myopia.

Stand with your legs as wide apart as possible, feet and knees open, torso straight, hands on the folds of the groin, under which pass the meridians of the liver. Inhale. As you exhale, do a knee bend on your right knee, turning your upper body (without bending it) toward your outstretched left leg. You should have your left foot turned inward and held completely flat to the ground. If possible, press the heel of your right foot on the ground as well. Your torso should remain as straight as possible.

Perform this same movement on the right, bending on your left knee (see Photos 192 and 193). Repeat the exercise at least three times on each side, concentrating on the tension that can be felt on the inside of the leg along the meridian of the liver.

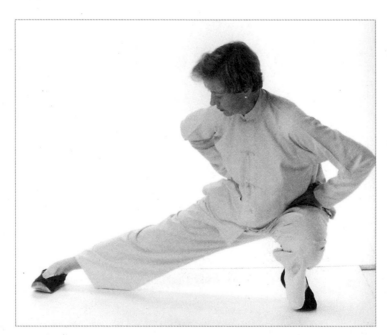

Photo 192

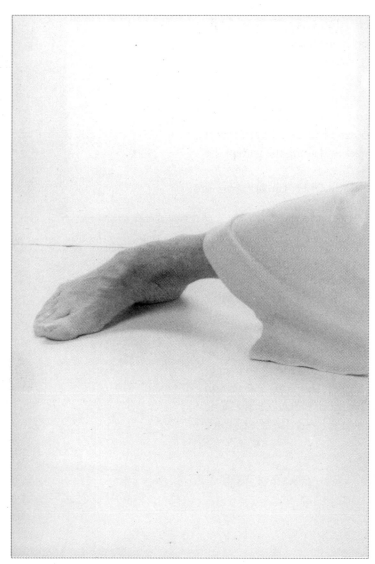

Photo 193

Gall Bladder Meridian

The gall bladder, a yang organ connected to the yin liver, is classified by Chinese medicine as among the "curious" viscera and is nourished by energy from the special meridians—in particular from the daimai meridian, which encircles the waist. Thanks to this link with the daimai meridian, the gall bladder is tied into the essential energy, which is carried by the special meridians. According to traditional Chinese medicine, the psychological capacity to "struggle through" problems is dependent on the gall bladder.

This exercise is also useful in case of aches and pains in the legs and knees and along the path of the meridian.

See Photos 194 to 196 for this exercise. As you inhale, take a step forward with your left foot, pressing the heel to the ground and turning the front of the foot outward. At the same time, raise your arms and your interlaced hands toward the left and up over your head. Shift your body weight onto your left leg, resting your right foot as much as possible on the front side of its fourth toe, where the meridian terminates. Your body is now twisted. Concentrate on the tension you feel along the meridian. Stop twisting when you can catch a glimpse of your right foot as you look over your left shoulder. Exhale and return to your original position. Proceed in the same way on the right and repeat the exercise at least three times on each side.

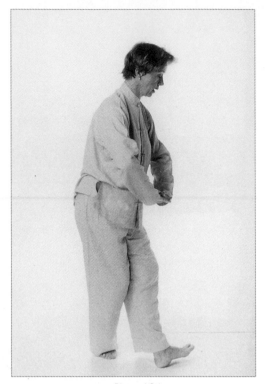

Photo 194

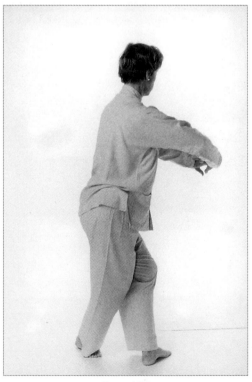

Photo 195

How to Stay in Great Shape

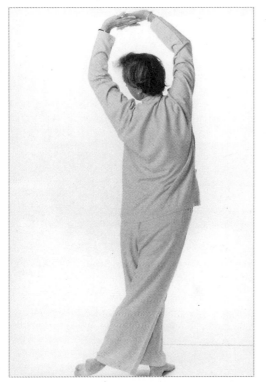

Photo 196

Heart and Small Intestine Meridians

For this exercise see Photos 197 and 198. Sit down with your knees spread wide and your feet joined sole to sole. Now fold the laced fingers of your hands over the tips of your feet, so that you enclose them, and pull them slightly upward as you inhale. As you exhale, bend your upper body forward, bringing your forehead close to your feet and jutting your bent elbows in front of your legs. Repeat this exercise several times, concentrating on the tension you feel along the routes of the two meridians of the heart and the small intestine as you exhale.

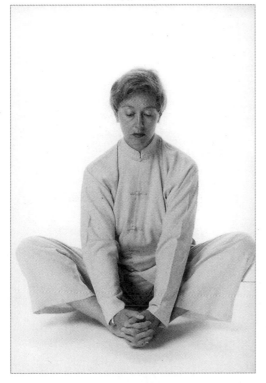

Photo 197

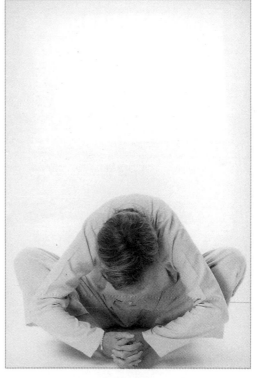

Photo 198

5
Qigong and Sexuality

Sexuality in Traditional Chinese Medicine

The importance of a harmonious sex life to physical and psychic well-being has always been emphasized in ancient texts of medicine and philosophy. In ancient China this subject was not a matter of ethical or religious taboos; man joining with woman was the symbol of the fundamental principle of the universe: the union of yin and yang. Two thousand years ago the great philosopher Confucious said, "Hunger and sexual desire are inherent to human nature." In the ancient *Li Ji* (Book of Rites), another sage declared, "The principal desires are to eat and make love."

To the Chinese, sex not only was a natural activity but because of its tremendous importance to physical and psychic life was utilized as a therapeutic exercise. The first mention of this is found in a book from the Han epoch written on tablets of bamboo, *He Yin Yang* (The Union of Yin and Yang), found in a tomb in Mawangdui. "Sexual intercourse," it

reads, "can make energy and blood circulate throughout the body and benefits all the inner organs." Another author of antiquity, Ge Hong, stated in his work *Bao Pu Ze,* "The sexual act is indispensable to both man and woman. If desire is suffocated, illness arises and life is shortened." Later, during the Tang epoch, the doctor Sun Se Miao confirmed: "Man cannot do without woman nor woman without man. Lack of sexual pleasure wearies the spirit and harms the health."

It is significant that already in the most ancient texts there is mention of *woman* and the necessity of satisfying her. In the Taoist treatise *Dong Xuanzi*, we read: "Before ejaculation, even if the man desires it, one must make sure that the woman has enjoyed pleasure."

Almost all of the erotic manuals and texts of Chinese medicine that deal with this subject affirm the importance of awakening desire through foreplay and erotic games: kisses, caresses, and massage. The art of lovemaking and sexually pleasing a woman was already practiced in China three thousand years ago at a time when our female ancestors in Europe suffered from brutal couplings on demand.

Ancient China was learned in sexology, by which was understood respect for both man and woman and for nature and the principle of moderation. In one treatise (*Li Fang Lei Ju*—A Collection of Prescriptions—by Jin Limeng), we read, "Sexuality can be either beneficial or harmful. He who understands how to use it will live long and healthfully, while he who abuses it may die prematurely. Sperm is important to the man, it is a vital energy that should not be scattered foolishly, while blood is important to the woman. The accumulation of sperm renders desire ardent. And when blood circulation is activated, the woman can more readily conceive a child."

These texts place few limits on sexual activity in women, but they advise men to limit, in reasonable measure and according to their age, not the frequency of sexual encounters—which they encourage—but the number of actual ejaculations. How can this be done? Following find a summary of some of the methods put forward in the ancient manuals.

The Chinese Art of Making Love

In a tomb discovered in 1974 in Mawangdui, dating from the Han epoch, a book written on tablets of bamboo was found: *Tian Xia Zhi Dao Tan* (The Way of the World), in which the author describes the various difficulties that may arise during sexual intercourse and provides methods to follow for their alleviation.

The Seven Dangers. The following are dangers to be avoided:

1. "Internal closure": During the sexual act, the man's seminal duct becomes obstructed and pain is severe.
2. "Emanation of the yin outward": This condition manifests as heavy perspiration, often leading to colds.
3. "Overindulgence": This exhausts sperm and weakens vital energy.

4. "Impotence": Psychological factors or weakness in the internal organs can cause impotence.
5. "Boredom": This can provoke dizziness and breathlessness during intercourse.
6. "Blind alley": Forced penetration of the penis undermines a successful outcome during intercourse and harms the health of the woman, who should instead be approached with sweet preliminaries.
7. "Loss of energy": Also known as premature ejaculation, this shortens the duration of intercourse and disperses the man's vital energy.

The Eight Methods. Faced with these dangers, we can turn to the "eight methods," which are simply relaxation and breath-control exercises with the purpose of bringing the couple to a good sexual understanding.

1. "Circulate the qi": Sit down on the bed with your back straight and contract your anus while mentally bringing the energy down into the genital organs.
2. "Emit the secretion": Breathe deeply and relax the tension in your muscles to facilitate the secretion of love's liquids.
3. "Wait for the right moment": Do not rush through things; do not skip the preliminaries, those caresses and erotic games so necessary for physical and mental extension. True sex begins only when both partners burn with desire and their minds and bodies are ready.
4. "Accumulate the qi": Contract the anus during sexual engagement and continue to concentrate on the descent of energy into the genitals.
5. "Stimulate the secretions": Penetration should be sweet, its movements gentle and harmonious, alternately long and short to stimulate the vaginal secretions of the woman and bring her gradually to pleasure. The woman should evince the "five reactions": when vital energy reaches the heart, her face becomes red; when vital energy reaches the liver, she looks wildly in all directions; when vital energy reaches the

lungs, she says nothing more and her nose grows damp; when it arrives at the spleen, she rubs her neck against the neck of her man; and when it reaches the kidneys, the vagina is lubricated and opens. At this point, the woman is ready.

6. "Maintain the qi": Withdraw the penis while it is still hard to avoid finishing too soon.
7. "Wait until the qi is at its peak and the woman has experienced pleasure."
8. If at the moment of ejaculation the man does not wish to release his vital energy, he must contract his anus, open his eyes very wide, squeeze his hands into fists, and concentrate on the qi energy, mentally directing it up the spine to his brain.

By following these "eight methods" and avoiding the "seven dangers," the two lovers can easily attain sexual happiness and long life.

Commonsense Rules: Being in Harmony with Yourself, Your Partner, and Your Environment

The ancient texts advise against sexual intercourse in certain situations. Among these are a full stomach; drunkenness; a state of anger, weariness, or fear; an emotional extreme of either joy or sorrow; after a bath during a fever; or when the woman is menstruating or has just given birth. In other words, sexual intercourse is discouraged in situations of physical or affective imbalance. Since the function of the internal organs is strictly linked to the "seven emotions," excess emotion combined with the nervous excitement of sex can damage the health.

To the Chinese the human being is an integral part of nature; therefore any change in climate exerts an influence on the organs of the body. For this reason, a relaxing environment and a mild climate enhance the quality of a person's sex life. Atmospheric excesses, such as intense cold or scorching heat, unbalance the yin and yang energies and encourage the infiltration of "perverse breaths" in the internal organs. Abstention from sex is advised, then, in conditions of storm, violent wind, intense cold or heat, heavy rain, and eclipses of the sun or moon. In such cases, nature itself is "out of sync."

As always, the best way is the way of moderation. Longevity depends on the manner in which sexuality is managed: Moderation leads to long life and good health. Men are particularly at risk if they disperse their vital energies through too-frequent ejaculations, exhausting the energy of the kidneys. In this case they will soon observe in themselves the signs of premature aging, such as impotence, loss of hearing and memory, and early graying.

These same ancient texts give advice regarding the frequency of sexual relations for women: "A woman in her twenties can have intercourse every two days; in her thirties, every three days; in her forties, every four days; in her fifties, every five days. After sixty years of age it is better to abstain." This advice, however, was written by men!

The Play of Sexual Yin and Yang Energies

At the base of all these recommendations and beliefs lies a sexual education founded on the theory of yin and yang.

To increase his own energy and to secure himself health and long life, the man must set in motion the deepest yin of the woman (present in the lubricating liquids of the vagina) and soak himself in them during intercourse. At the moment of orgasm, the woman also sets free her own yang, thus allowing the man to take possession of it.

It is understandable, following this premise, that according to tradition the more frequent his relations with young, "fresh" women, the more the man enriches his own vitality—always on the condition that he does not ejaculate but mentally directs the energy to his brain at the peak of excitement. One need only think of the many concubines of the Chinese emperors.

In the same way, the woman absorbs the yang energy of the man. Not chauvinist in this regard, the Chinese cite the example of the empress Wu Tze Tian, who at an advanced age still appeared very young, thanks to her large "consumption" of young courtiers. It is for this reason that the texts warn men not to make love with women older and more experienced than they are—these women could rob them of their yang!

Key Functions of the Body for Female Sexuality

Blood and the Yang Qi of the Kidneys. According to traditional Chinese medicine, blood is composed of nutritive elements and organic liquid. These substances are formed by the transformation of food, absorbed and digested by the stomach and spleen. The nutrient effect of the blood is manifested as muscle tone and good health. In cases of deficiency or loss of blood, this function is reduced, leading to pathological phenomena. Blood also has a noble function: It is the material support of the activities of the spirit.

Since energy and blood are indispensable to growth and reproduction, a deficiency of either one creates disturbances in sexual functioning. To treat such disturbances qigong therefore works on the energy of the two organs most closely linked to the blood—the heart and the liver—and on the energy of the kidneys, the repository of sexual vigor.

The Heart: The cardiac impulse is fundamental. If it is weak, it adversely affects sexual functioning.

The Liver: The liver is responsible for various key functions that affect sexuality. It tones muscles, filters and stores blood, directs venous circulation, regulates the energetic mechanism, stimulates digestion, and encourages good humor. A certain reserve of blood is stored in the liver to be used in emergencies (hemorrhage, for example), and this is the blood that is freed to fill the penis at the moment of erection. Ovulation and menstruation in women and erection and ejaculation in men are closely connected to the health of the liver.

The Kidneys: The kidneys conserve prenatal or "preceding sky" energy, inherited from the parents, and postnatal or "following sky" energy, extracted from food. The kidneys govern growth, the development of bones and marrow, reproduction and the genital organs, and almost the entire metabolic system. The yin of the kidneys nourishes various organs; their yang exerts a stimulant effect on the whole organism.

The yang qi of the kidneys plays a predominant role in sexual activity: It constitutes "the fire of life," the source and motive force of vital human energy. If the yang qi of the kidneys is depleted, women may experience disturbances of the uterus (such as uterine bleeding), fatigue, lower back pain, and a decrease in libido; men may suffer from impotence, premature ejaculation, and seminal loss. Both men and women in this situation may complain of stiffness in the arms and legs, a tendency to feel cold, nightsweats, weakness, and premature aging.

The yang qi of the kidneys stimulates the physiology of the sex act, conditions the production of sperm, and regulates the menstrual cycle.

Men who indulge in an immoderate sex life exhaust the yang qi of the kidneys, which according to Chinese medicine is the only energy that cannot be augmented. It must therefore be preserved and improved qualitatively with the massages and exercises of qigong.

Qigong and Sexuality

Massages to Tone and Stimulate Sexual Energy

In erotic Chinese texts massages form an integral part of foreplay. They offer a reciprocal and pleasureable kind of invigoration, a prelude to more exciting play. Certain of the digital manipulations and massages can also be used for therapeutic purposes.

For all of the following exercises, massage each point indicated for one or two minutes in a circular motion or by vertical pressure with the tip of the finger. If it seems too complicated to you to massage these points one by one, you can use the following method, since most of the points are located on the median line of the torso: Massage your partner's back, first from the coccyx up the spine (Du Mai meridian) to the neck, then 1½ cuns on either side of the spine (bladder meridian). Then massage his or her stomach along the median line of the body from the navel down to the pubis (Ren Mai meridian) and in the same direction 2 cuns from this axis (stomach meridian). These massages are both relaxing and invigorating!

Some other "love points" are as follows:

• *Huiyin* (1 RM): halfway between the anus and the vagina or testicles (see Figure 14). It is also indicated for disturbances in the menstrual cycle.

• *Baihui* (20 DM): on the top of the head, at the intersection of the median line of the cranium and the line that connects to the tips of both ears (see Figure 8). This is the most invigorating point for yang.

• *Zhongwan* (12 RM): on the abdomen, 4 cuns above the navel on the longitudinal medial axis of the trunk (see Figure 15). It is indicated for sexual disturbances due to gastric dysfunction.

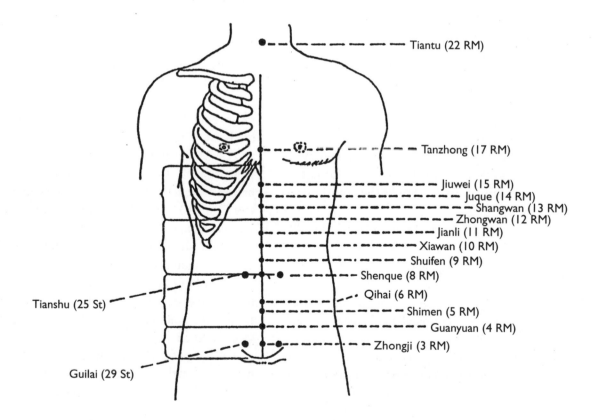

Figure 15: The points of the abdomen

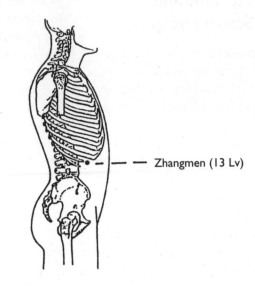

Figure 16: The Zhangmen point on the floating rib

• *Zhangmen* (13 Lv): just below the free-floating tip of the eleventh rib (see Figure 16). This activates blood circulation, invigorates the spleen, and unblocks the meridians.

• *Shenque* (8 RM): in the center of the navel (see Figure 15). This massage is indicated for sterility in women, for weakness of the kidneys, and for gastric and intestinal disturbances. Stroke the point or heat it with moxa.

• *Tianshu* (25 St): 2 cuns from the navel, laterally on both sides (see Figure 15). This massage regularizes vital energy, cures sexual problems in women, and regulates menstruation.

• *Qihai* (6 RM): 1½ cuns below the navel (see Figure 15). Indicated for irregularity of the menstrual cycle and for leukorrhea.

• *Guanyuan* (4 RM): 3 cuns below the navel (see Figure 15). This strengthens sexual functioning. It is also indicated for menstrual irregularity and dysmenorrhea.

• *Zhongji* (3 RM): 4 cuns below the navel (see Figure 15). It invigorates yang and is useful for menstrual disturbances and itching of the vulva.

• *Xinshu* (15 B): on the back, 1½ cuns to the outside of the space between the fifth and sixth thoracic vertebrae (see Figure 8). This is the point of the heart; it regularizes the blood and vital energy and calms the spirit.

• *Geshu* (17 B): 1½ cuns to the side of the space between the seventh and eighth thoracic vertebrae (see Figure 8). This point connects with the cardiovascular system. It invigorates the kidneys, regulates the blood, stimulates circulation, and disperses excessive sanguinary heat.

• *Shenshu* (23 B): 1½ cuns to the side of the space between the second and third vertebrae (see Figure 8). It is the point connected to the kidneys and invigorates their yang qi.

• *Mingmen* (4 DM): on the posterior median axis of the trunk at the level of the waist, between the apophyses of the second and third lumbar vertebrae (see Figure 8). This strengthens sexual potency (massage the *Mingmen* of your partner!) and acts as an anti-inflammatory for the uterine canal and the vagina.

Qigong and Sexuality

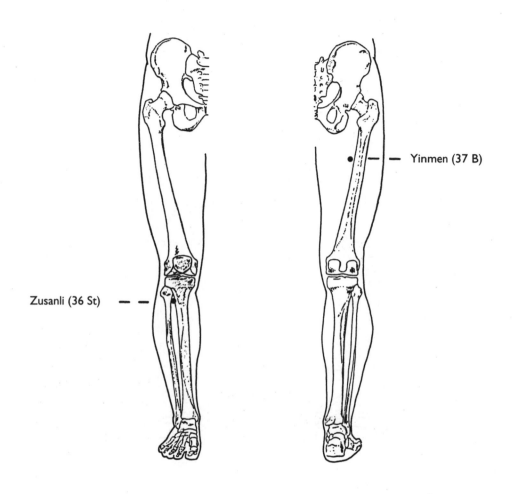

Zusanli (36 St) — —

Yinmen (37 B)

Figure 17: Some points on the front and back of the leg

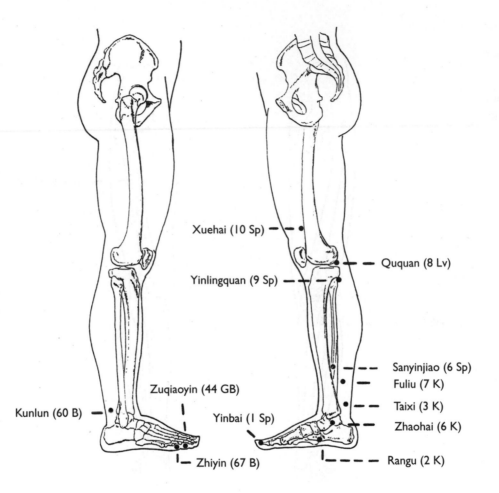

Figure 18: Some points on the inner and outer sides of the leg and foot

Xuehai (10 Sp)

Ququan (8 Lv)

Yinlingquan (9 Sp)

Sanyinjiao (6 Sp)
Fuliu (7 K)

Zuqiaoyin (44 GB)

Taixi (3 K)

Kunlun (60 B)

Zhaohai (6 K)

Yinbai (1 Sp)

Zhiyin (67 B)

Rangu (2 K)

- *Yaoyan* (21 Ext): over the kidneys below the apophyses of the fourth lumbar vertebra, 3½ cuns to the side of the spine (see Figure 8). This point invigorates the energy of the kidneys and prevents sexual problems.

- *Jianshi* (5 P): 3 cuns above the fold of the wrist, between the tendons (see Figure 11). This has a calming effect on the body's internal heat and is indicated for disturbances in the menstrual cycle and for leukorrhea.

- *Yuji* (10 Lu): on the palm side of the hand, in the center of the pad at the base of the thumb, halfway to the first metacarpal (see Figure 11). It disperses excess heat and prevents dispersion of the yin. It is also indicated for problems of the vulva and sexual disturbances caused by weakness of the spleen and lack of yin.

- *Zusanli* (36 St): 3 cuns below the lower edge of the kneecap and a finger's width to the outside of the anterior tibial crest (see Figure 17). This is the point of invigoration par excellence for all the functions of the body.

- *Sanyinjiao* (6 Sp): on the inside of the leg, 3 cuns above the inner side of the ankle bone and behind the inner edge of the tibia (see Figure 18). This strengthens the yin and invigorates the blood and vital energy; it is indicated for sexual disturbances and breech birth.

- *Taixi* (3 K): halfway between the inner tip of the ankle bone and Achilles' tendon (see Figure 18). It invigorates the yin of the kidneys and is indicated for disturbances of the menstrual cycle and sexual dysfunction.

- *Taichong* (3 Lv): on the upper surface of the foot in the hollow of the first metatarsal space (see Figure 12). It is indicated for disturbances of the menstrual cycle and for mastitis and invigorates the blood in the liver.

How to Overcome Frigidity

If a woman feels no pleasure during sexual intercourse, if she remains indifferent or is unable to reach orgasm, psychological problems are the most usual culprits. The first step is to accept your own body just as it is and not to be ashamed of your pleasure. The exercises described in Chapter 2 are helpful for this.

But physiological causes for frigidity are also acknowledged in traditional Chinese medicine, and these can be cured by massages, exercises, and therapeutic sounds. See the second section of Chapter 3 for instructions on how to practice these sounds.

The principal physiological causes of frigidity are:

Deficiency of Yang Qi in the Kidneys

Symptoms. Indifference, inability to feel sexual pleasure, a sensation of cold, pain in the genital organs, anxiety, aches and pains in the lower back and knees, irregular menstruation, and a sensation of cold in the abdomen.

Treatment.

- Practice the sounds "Chui" and "Hong" 20 times a day to reinvigorate the kidneys, as well as practicing the sounds "Ssss" and Ni," which are linked to the lungs (the lungs are "the mother" of the kidneys, to which they transmit energy according to the model of the five elements).

- Massage the kidney meridian, which runs along the legs, being particularly sure to massage the points *Yongquan* (1 K, see Figure 5), *Taixi, Zhaohai,* and *Fuliu* (3, 6, and 7 K, see Figure 18 and, at the back of the book, the figure showing the kidney meridian). In addition, press the points *Shenshu* (23 B) and *Jingmen* (25 GB) on the back (see Figure 8).

- Do the exercises listed at the end of this chapter.

Weakness of the Heart and Spleen

Symptoms. Indifference, mental fatigue, melancholy, pale face, loss of appetite, constipation, menstrual irregularity, breathlessness.

Treatment.

- Practice the therapeutic sounds "Ke" and "Haa" to strengthen the heart and "Chui" and "Hong" to harmonize heart and kidneys. In addition, practice the sounds "Hu" and "Mei" to invigorate the spleen and stomach.

• Massage along the path of the heart meridian from the chest to the tips of the fingers. Also massage along the spleen meridian on the inside of the leg from the foot on up, being especially sure to massage the points *Yinbai* (1 Sp, see Figure 12), *Sanyinjiao, Yinlingquan,* and *Xuehai* (6, 9, and 10 Sp, see Figure 18).

• Press the following points: *Juque* (14 RM, see Figure 7), *Shengmen* (7 H, see Figure 11), *Pishu* (20 B, see Figure 8), and *Zusanli* (36 St, see Figure 17).

• Do the exercises listed at the end of this chapter.

Stasis in the Energy of the Liver

Symptoms. Inability to enjoy sexual relations, anxiety, bad moods, agitation, frequent anger, dysmenorrhea, disturbances in the menstrual cycle.

Treatment.

• Practice the sounds "Xu" and "Pa," which are linked to the liver, the regulator of emotions, and also the sounds of the heart, "Ke" and "Haa," to harmonize heart and liver.

• Press the following points: *Ganshu* (18 B, see Figure 8), *Qimen* (14 Lv, see Figure 7), *Taichong* (3 Lv, see Figure 12), and *Ququan* (8 Lv, see Figure 13).

• Practice the exercises listed below.

Exercises

It is recommended that women with problems of frigidity take a warm footbath every evening and that at bedtime their partner give them the following massage, which activates blood circulation.

Massage

Massage the dorsal and lumbar vertebrae, making sure to use acupressure in the spaces between them. Then provide a circular massage in the region of the coccyx with the two palms of the hands, one placed above the other. Stroke the muscles alongside the spine, being sure to press the points *Shenshu, Zhishi,* and *Ciliao* (23, 52, and 32 B, see Figure 8). Spend an equal amount of time massaging the legs and feet, being

sure to press the vital points *Yinmen* (37 B, see Figure 17), *Sanyinjiao* (6 Sp, see Figure 18), *Rangu* (2 K, see Figure 18), and *Yongquan* (1 K, see Figure 5).

Relaxing Breathing Exercises

The exercise of the "pink balloon" described in Chapter 3 is recommended for relaxation. In addition to the "pink balloon," you may wish to perform the following relaxation exercise:

Seated on the floor (see Photos 199 to 201), put your palms down behind your back and spread your legs. As you inhale, turn the tips of your feet outward while leaning your torso and head backward. As you exhale, turn the tips of your feet inward while straightening out your torso and letting your head drop forward.

Then, still seated with your legs stretched out, stretch your arms out in front of your chest as you exhale. As you inhale, fold them back toward your hips while contracting your anus. Repeat at least nine times.

Contraindication: Abstain from this exercise during menstruation.

Toning and Invigorating Exercises

Women who wish to improve sexual functioning can tone and invigorate energy by a series of auto-massages and exercises. Following are several that are simple and easy to do. For more complex exercises, refer to Mantak Chia's book, *Taoist Secrets of Love.*

Massaging the Breasts. Using only three fingers, massage around your nipples with a circular motion, moving from the inside to the outside, to stimulate the endocrine glands (three to five minutes each day).

Drawing on the Energy of the Ovaries. The time in your cycle between the end of menstruation and the onset of ovulation is when the energy of your ovaries is at the peak of its yang. During this period, by using a technique of focused breathing, you can draw on this yang energy and make it circulate by doing the following:

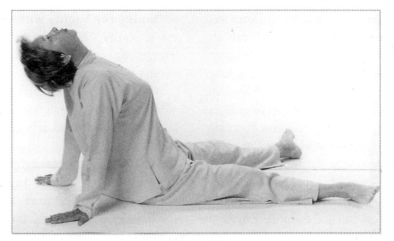

Photo 199

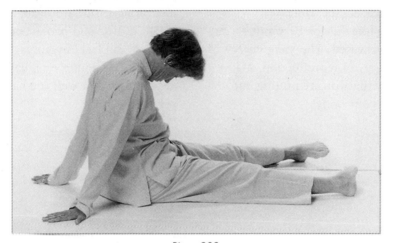

Photo 200

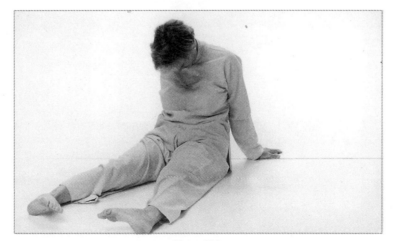

Photo 201

Sit in a chair with your back straight and your feet on the ground and rest the palms of your hands on your ovaries with your fingers pointing toward your pubis. Close your eyes and place your tongue against your upper palate. First perform a series of abdominal respirations, puffing the abdomen out as you inhale and lightly contracting it as you exhale, concentrating the whole time on the sensation of warm energy in your ovaries. Once you feel the warmth, mentally diffuse it throughout the lower womb. Then while inhaling and contracting your anus, push this energy even lower toward your perineum and from there make it climb up your spine until it reaches your brain. As you exhale, mentally guide the energy down the front of your body until it reaches the dantian.

Practice breathing like this for 10 minutes a day during the period indicated. The yang energy of the ovaries is the energy of reproduction, so it is a very powerful energy that you are putting into circulation throughout your body.

Toning the Vagina with an Egg. Since remotest antiquity Chinese women have used the egg exercise to tone and strengthen the muscles of the vagina.

The egg should be made of marble or polished stone, neither too small nor too large, and should be adequately disinfected or boiled before use. The procedure is as follows:

Stand with your legs slightly apart, introduce the egg into your vagina, and then position your closed fists at the level of the groin. As you inhale, contract the muscles that close the orifice of the vagina and continue the contraction so that you are actually pushing the egg upward. Allow it to slowly descend, then bring it upward again. When you are out of breath, exhale and pause, concentrating on the energy you can feel in your vagina. Practice this exercise 3 to 10 minutes each day. (Then let your partner discover how well you have learned to use your pelvic muscles!)

6
Common Physical Problems of Women

Maintaining Healthy Bones and Joints: The "Golden Marrow" Exercises

In the period of the climacteric, hormone production slows down and some hormones that have the function of providing and directing calcium drop out altogether. Once this process of decalcification is set in motion, the bones become fragile. But certain exercises drawn from traditional Chinese medicine that invigorate the energy of the kidneys can halt the drop in hormone production. The kidneys play an important role in the production of certain vital hormones, among which are adrenaline, aldosterone, cortisol, and steroidal hormones. According to recent studies, practitioners of qigong maintain a fairly high percentage of these hormones in the blood no matter what their age.

First let us examine some exercises from the "Golden Marrow" series, conceived precisely to prevent and cure aging of the joints and bones. I present a few of the most efficacious exercises, which should

be performed faithfully every day. Persons already afflicted with arthritis will notice a marked improvement after two months of practice.

In Chinese the "Golden Marrow" exercises are called *Xi Sui Yin Jin,* that is to say, "Washing the Bone Marrow and Fortifying the Tendons." According to tradition, they were invented by the Indian monk Bodhidharma, called by the Chinese Da Mo, who in the fifth century A.D. brought the teachings of Buddha to China. On his way back to India, Bodhidharma stayed in the monastery of Shaolin, which later became famous for its school of martial arts, and during his stay he taught the monks this series of "Golden Marrow" exercises, as well as the "Classic of the Tendons" (the *Yi Jin Jing*), a series of stretching exercises useful for recovering flexibility in the joints after hours of sitting meditation.

The author of the following exercises, Ma Li Tang, learned the series from his teacher Pu Zhao in 1932, and later from Wu Che, a monk in the monastery of Wu Tai Shan in northeastern China, who gave him an ancient manuscript containing a version of the "Golden Marrow" from the ninth century. Basing his work on this manuscript, Ma Li Tang created his own abbreviated series, completing it with some longevity exercises practiced in China since the Sung dynasty in the eleventh century.

The practice of these longevity exercises has been constant in China. During the Sung dynasty the poet Su She and the doctor Shen Kuo had already acknowledged face massage, digital acupressure, and so forth as "doors to longevity," which is how they presented them. During the Ming dynasty in the sixteenth century the doctor Lang Lian recommended that people repeat simple daily exercises such as tapping the teeth, massaging the head, and rolling the eyes.

The "Golden Marrow" is a combination of various ancient versions, but Ma Li Tang adapted and simplified them to compose a series of twenty-three easy exercises. The "Golden Marrow" is a holistic method that combines automassage, breath control, and muscle and tendon stretches while nourishing and strengthening bone marrow. Although movement and automassage are the central aspects of these exercises, mental concentration, directing and guiding the flow of the qi energy, is also very important.

The purpose of the exercises is to expel pathogens from the bones and tendons, improving blood flow and the circulation of qi and rendering the body more flexible in a few weeks of daily practice. As for their effect on the marrow, the mechanism is internal: Stretching the tendons results in an increase in blood flow and qi in the bones, thus improving the biological exchange that allows the marrow to be oxygenated. By means of these exercises, then, we are seeking to actuate a true regeneration of the marrow, important not only to the health of the bones—the Chinese say that if the marrow is in good condition, the brain functions well.

Following you will find some different ways you can practice these exercises.

Breathing. Inhale and exhale through the nose, concentrating your attention on the qi energy flowing through your body, guided by your mind. To augment the effect of energetic circulation, follow this method: Let your abdomen swell out as you inhale and contract your abdominal muscles as you exhale. In this way, according to a Chinese saying, "Qi arrives swiftly and illness vanishes."

Single and Serial Exercises. The exercises can be split according to the needs of the practitioner. It is best to repeat each exercise eight times (or a multiple of eight). As preventive treatment and to maintain good health, doing the entire series daily is recommended.

At the end of a series, or even of a single exercise, be sure to remember the fundamental rule of qigong: *Always* mentally bring the energy back to the dantian (see page 16 in Chapter 1). And at the beginning of each exercise, *always* assume the basic position.

The Basic Position. This is the basic position for almost all the exercises of qigong.

Stand straight with your feet apart so that they are in line with your shoulders, with your body weight evenly distributed over the entire surface of each foot. Your knees should be slightly flexed, your shoulders relaxed, your armpits soft and held slightly open, as if they were holding an egg. Hold your arms so that they fall naturally to the sides of your body, elbows not rigid but rounded.

Your back should be straight and your head erect, your chin pulled slightly in. Imagine your head attached to a string that runs from the point *Baihui* (20 DM, see Figure 8), located at the apex of the cranium, to the sky itself. Visualize an upside-down Y connecting the points *Yongquan* (1 K, under the soles of the feet, see Figure 5), *Huiyin* (1 RM, on the perineum, see Figure 14), and *Baihui*. Relax your face and clear your mind. Hold your pelvic basin horizontal: Imagine it as a bowl full of liquid that you must not spill. This position strengthens the muscles of the buttocks.

Breathe naturally from the abdomen; your chest should stay still. Place your tongue against your upper palate and close your lips. Cross your hands below your navel on the dantian zone, receptacle of energy (see Figure 9), right hand covered by the left for women, left hand covered by the right for men,

Common Physical Problems of Women

superimposing the two *Laogong* points (8 P, see Figure 11) in the center of the palms. Keep your eyes halfway closed and gaze directly to the front without focusing.

Start each exercise from this basic position and before beginning a series bring about the "silence of the body" by harmonizing breathing, mind, and body.

For the basic rules of acupressure, see the traditional Chinese medicine section in the Introduction.

Finger Rotation ("Golden Marrow")

This exercise helps restore agility to the wrists, combats osteoarthritis in the joints, and slows down memory loss. It activates the three yin and the three yang meridians of the hand. It can be a good adjuvant to therapy for Parkinson's disease, in which case the therapy should include all the "Golden Marrow" exercises as well as the use of therapeutic sound, in particular the sound "Chui." A practitioner of traditional Chinese medicine can also prescribe a special diet for treating Parkinson's disease.

See Photos 202 to 213, which illustrate this exercise. With your elbows bent, raise your two palms in front of you, open and turned toward your face. As you inhale, letting your abdomen fill and swell, fold down the fingers of both hands one by one, starting from the little fingers. Then make a complete rotation of the wrists so that your hands come together back to back. Continue the rotation so that your curled fingers face away from your body and roll your hands away from each other until the backs of your fists face your body. Exhale as, beginning with the index fingers, you extend the fingers of both hands. Inhale again as, beginning with the little fingers, you curl your hands into fists once more and roll your fists together back to back with your curled fingers facing your body. Continue the rotation and exhale as, beginning with the index fingers, you extend the fingers of both hands with your palms once more held open in front of you.

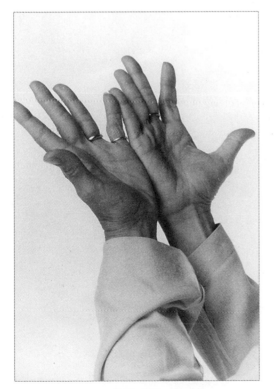

Photo 202

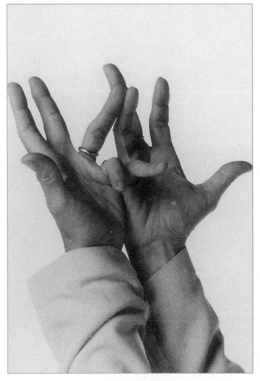

Photo 203

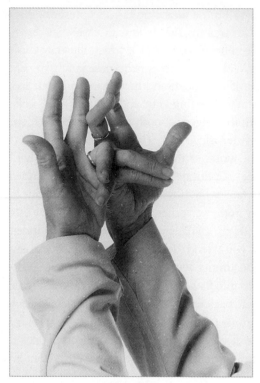

Photo 204

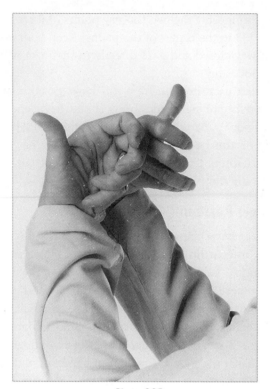

Photo 205

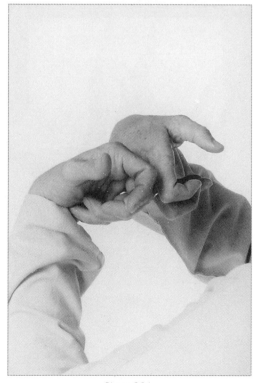

Photo 206

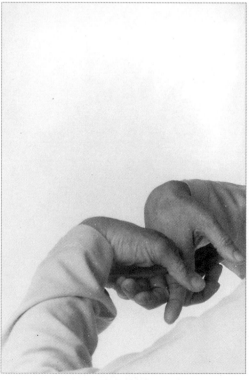

Photo 207

Common Physical Problems of Women

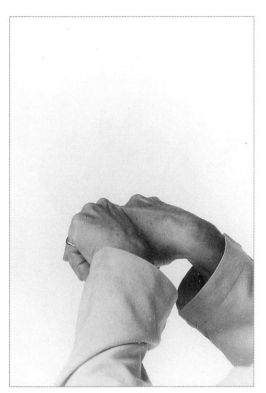

Photo 208

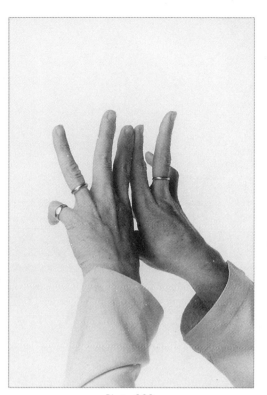

Photo 209

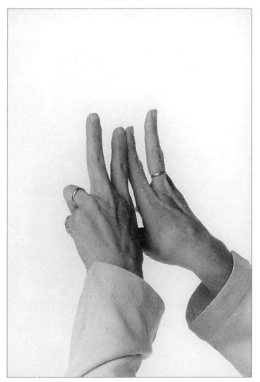

Photo 210

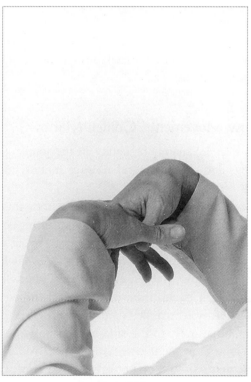

Photo 211

Common Physical Problems of Women

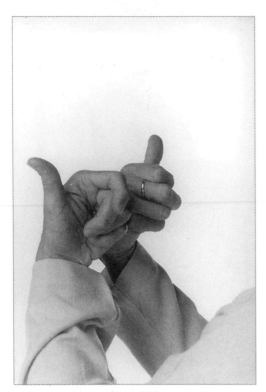

Photo 212

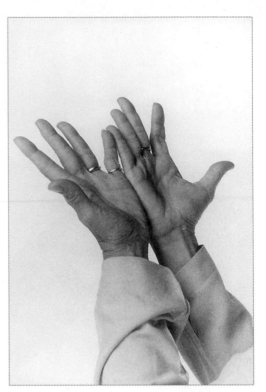

Photo 213

Concentrate your attention on keeping the rotation loose and soft. Repeat the exercise eight times, or for a multiple of eight.

Elbow Movement ("Golden Marrow")

This exercise maintains agility in the joints of the elbows and shoulders and restores motility in the arms.

See Photos 214 to 218, which illustrate this exercise. You can start either standing or sitting down. As you inhale, raise one arm in front of you, with the palm of the hand facing down, up to the level of the shoulder. As you exhale, bend your elbow and bring it backward with the palm turned up, until your wrist reaches your waist. Then let your arm fall naturally to the side of your body. Repeat the same movement with your other arm. These movements should be performed very slowly and your attention should be focused on your elbow.

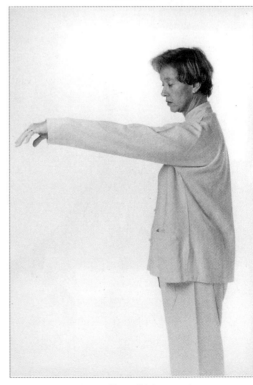

Photo 214

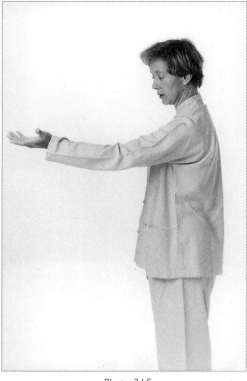

Photo 215

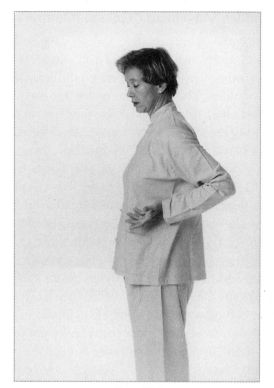

Photo 216

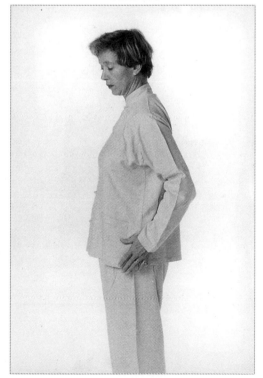

Photo 217

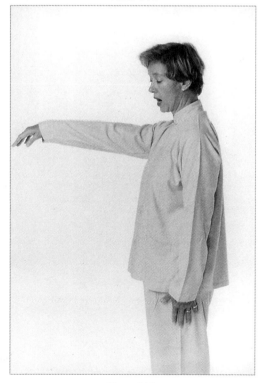

Photo 218

Shoulder Movement ("Golden Marrow")

This exercise is indicated for shoulder pain, bursitis, asthma, and pleurisy. Performed daily without fail for six months, it easily resolves motor disturbances of the shoulders. The exercise is divided into two parts.

Part One. As you inhale, raise your arms in front of you to the level of your shoulders with the palms of the hands facing down. As you exhale, draw back your elbows with the palms of your hands facing up. As you inhale again, raise your elbows, rotating them frontward until your hands are brought back to back at the level of the solar plexus (see Photos 219 to 225).

Then as you exhale, stretch your arms out in front of you and sweep them one to either side as if you were doing the breaststroke. When they touch each other behind your back, bring them forward again, bend your wrists and rotate them under your armpits, then lower your hands once more to the sides of your body.

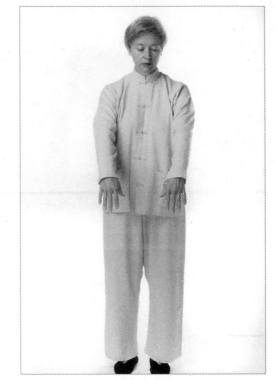

Photo 219

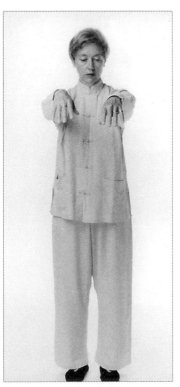

Photo 220

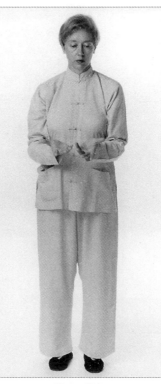

Photo 221

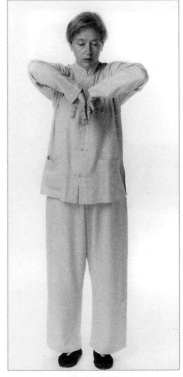

Photo 222

Common Physical Problems of Women

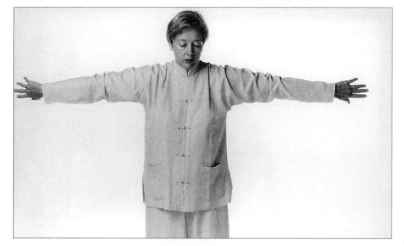

Photo 223

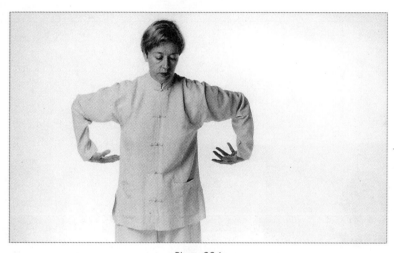

Photo 224

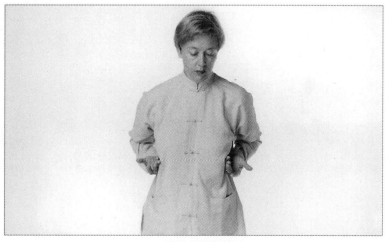

Photo 225

Part Two. As you inhale, lift your two hands back to back to the level of your solar plexus, raising your elbows. As you exhale, rotate your elbows to the back while opening your palms, thumbs touching your shoulders, and finish the movement by sliding your palms under your armpits and down the sides of your body (see Photos 226 to 230).

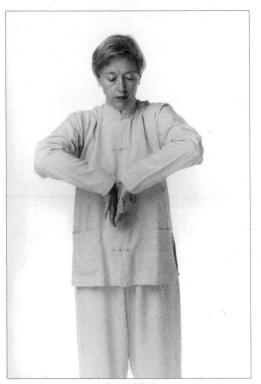

Photo 226

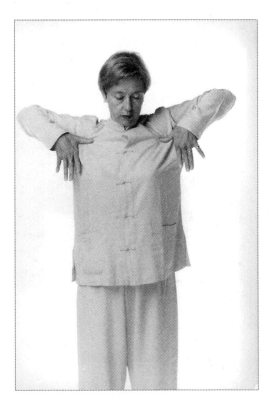

Photo 227

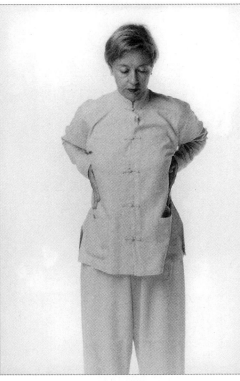

Photo 228

Common Physical Problems of Women

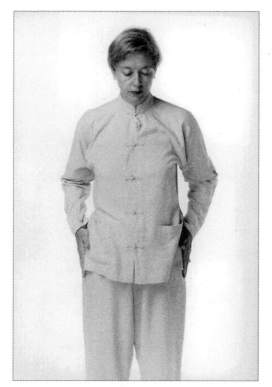

Photo 229

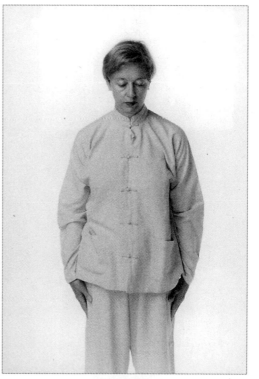

Photo 230

Stretching the Arms to Open the Breast ("Golden Marrow")

This exercise is indicated for pulmonary problems, since it augments respiratory capacity. Repeat it 8 to 64 times.

As you inhale, raise your arms in front of you to the level of your shoulders, open palms facing up. Now pull back your elbows, rotating your wrists at the level of the breast. As you exhale, push outward and to the sides with your open palms so that your arms perform a circle.

Now as you inhale again, move your arms backward and to the sides as if you were swimming, and when they touch each other behind your back, exhale, rotating your wrists and bringing your hands under your armpits, then sliding them down the sides of your body. See Photos 231 to 240.

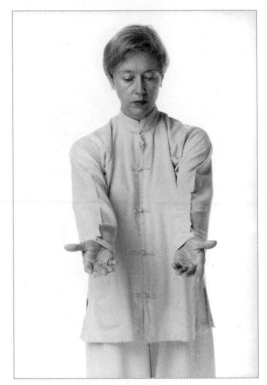

Photo 231

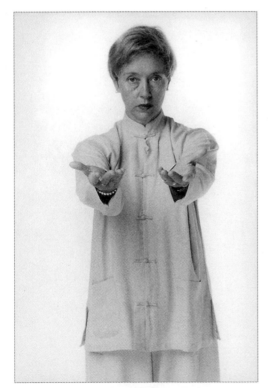

Photo 232

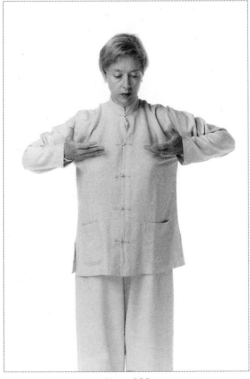

Photo 233

Common Physical Problems of Women

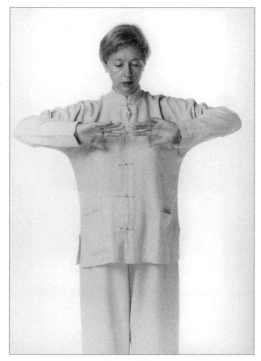

Photo 234

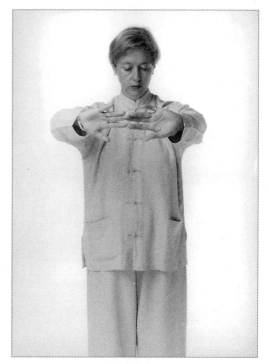

Photo 235

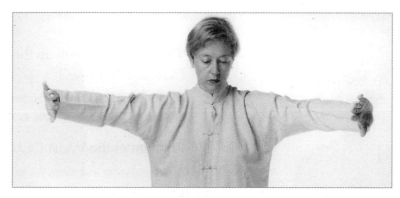

Photo 236

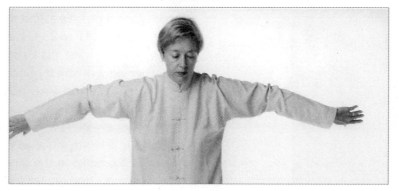

Photo 237

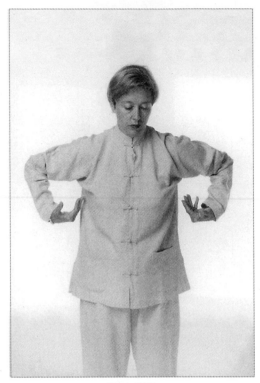

Photo 238

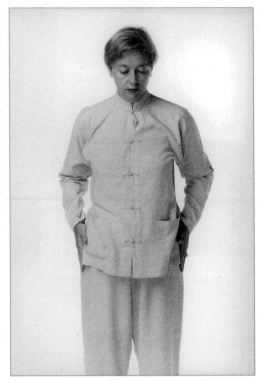

Photo 239

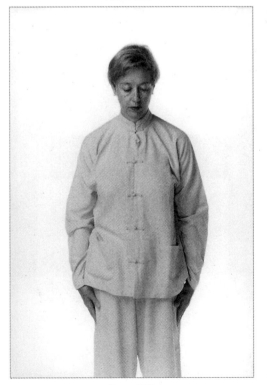

Photo 240

The Dragon Slithers up the Spine ("Golden Marrow")

See pages 26 to 28 in Chapter 2, accompanied by Photos 15 to 19, which illustrate this exercise.

Rotation of the Waist ("Golden Marrow")

This exercise is indicated for bone spurs, lower back pain, rheumatoid arthritis, hip joint problems, rigidity of the lower back and pelvis, kidney and gynecological problems, and impotence in men.

See Photos 241 to 244. Concentrating your attention on your waist, place the palms of your hands over your kidneys with the fingertips pointing down. As you inhale, thrust your pelvis forward, first toward the right foot, then toward the left foot, so that it describes a very wide half circle. As you exhale, make your pelvis describe an equally wide circle to the back. Continue in the same way, repeating the circle four times in a counterclockwise direction, then four times in a clockwise direction.

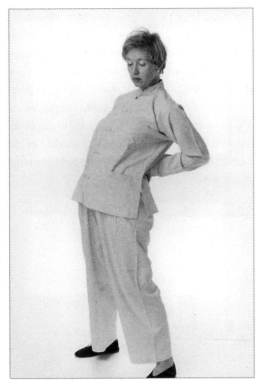

Photo 241

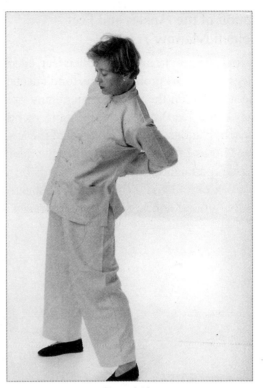

Photo 242

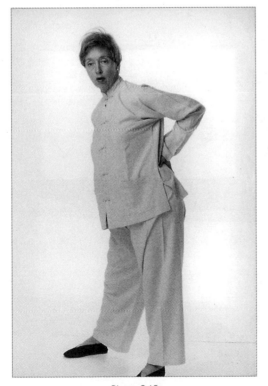

Photo 243

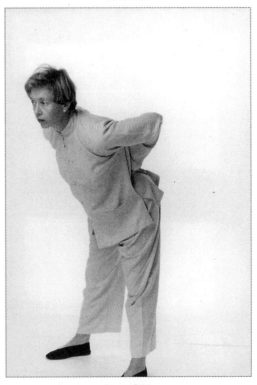

Photo 244

Common Physical Problems of Women

Rotation of the Ankles and Feet ("Golden Marrow")

This exercise is indicated for swollen feet, edema of the legs, and heart problems. It is fundamental because it works on the three yin meridians (spleen, kidneys, and liver) and the three yang meridians (stomach, bladder, and gall bladder) of the feet.

See Photos 245 to 249, which illustrate this exercise. Stand straight and with your hands on your hips work one foot at a time, lifting it slightly up from the ground and keeping the leg straight. Ro-

tate the foot four times in a counterclockwise direction, then four times in a clockwise direction in the following manner: As you inhale, flex the tip of the foot up toward the leg and rotate it so that it points first outward, then inward. Then, as you exhale, point the tip of the foot downward. Weak or elderly persons can do the exercise sitting or even lying down if they wish. If you are unable to move your ankle correctly, have someone gently manipulate it for you.

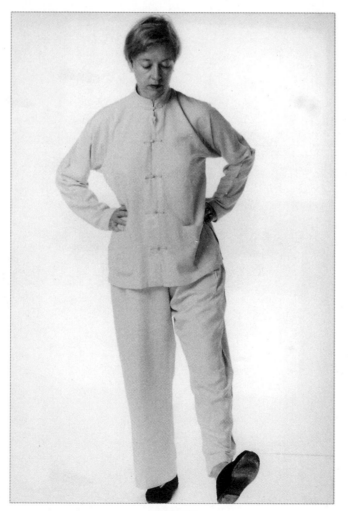

Photo 245

Common Physical Problems of Women

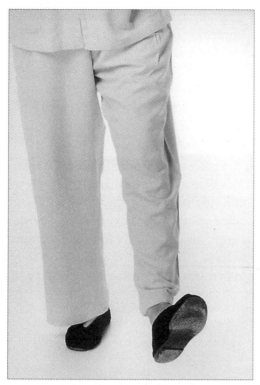

Photo 246

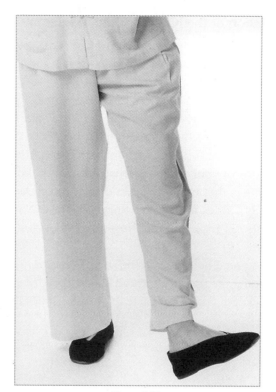

Photo 247

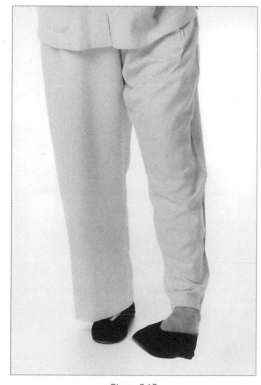

Photo 248

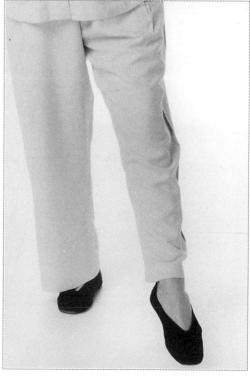

Photo 249

Common Physical Problems of Women

Rotation of the Knees ("Golden Marrow")

This exercise is indicated for problems of the knee joint or meniscus and for disturbances of the kidneys.

See Photos 250 to 253. Place the palms of your hands so that the *Laogong* point (8 P, see Figure 6) is in contact with the middle of your kneecaps. Concentrate your full attention on your knees. Arrange the tips of your fingers so that they touch the following points around your knees: thumb on *Xuehai* (10 Sp), index and middle fingers on the two *Xiyan* points (52 Ext), and ring finger on *Dubi* (35 St, see Figure 19).

As you inhale, pull up on your kneecaps, firmly grasping the points indicated above; then, bending both knees, manually rotate them in a counterclock-wise direction. Exhale and release the pressure of your fingers as you return to your initial position, with your legs straight, and press on your kneecaps with the center of the palm of your hands. Repeat the rotation four times counterclockwise (invigoration) and four times clockwise (dispersion).

Closure

To conclude the "Golden Marrow" series, rub your hands together, visualizing the energy concentrating in the *Laogong* points (8 P, see Figure 6); then place your palms on your eyes, envisioning the energy flowing into them. Then conduct the energy back down to the dantian as your hands slide down your face, neck, and chest to finally cross over the dantian.

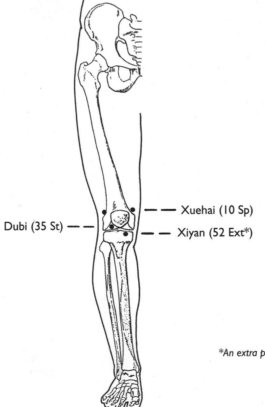

Dubi (35 St) — —   — — Xuehai (10 Sp)
                          — — Xiyan (52 Ext*)

An extra point that is not considered part of a meridian

Figure 19: Some points of the knee

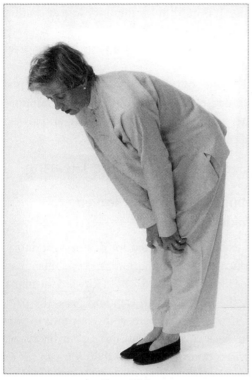

Photo 250

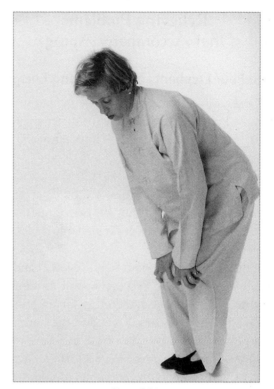

Photo 251

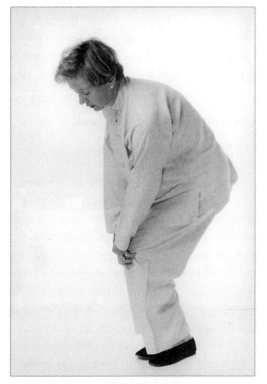

Photo 252

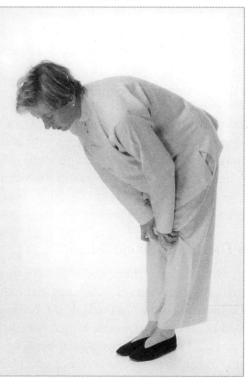

Photo 253

Relieving Problems that Accompany Aging

"The Four Elephants Nourish Yang Energy"

This exercise strengthens yang energy and invigorates the kidneys (and therefore the marrow and the brain). It is indicated in cases of impotence and nervous exhaustion.

Contraindications: Persons suffering from heart problems or high blood pressure should *not* do this exercise. It should also not be performed in the evening, since it stimulates yang energy, which can result in sleeplessness.

Stand straight with your heels together and the tips of your toes held as widely apart as possible. Bending your knees, descend as far as possible while holding your torso erect and the bottom of your pelvis tilted forward to erase the curve of the kidneys. Bring your arms out to form a circle in front of your body with the palms of your hands facing the dantian. Rest the tip of your tongue against your upper palate. Concentrate on the *Mingmen* point (4 DM, see Figure 8) between the second and third lumbar vertebrae, particularly when you are exhaling.

In this position, which encourages the opening of the *Mingmen* and the kidney meridian, repeat a series of abdominal respirations: While inhaling, push the abdomen out; while exhaling, contract the abdominal muscles, mentally directing energy to the kidneys.

Repeat the exercise with maximum concentration, first for 3 minutes, then gradually lengthening the practice time up to 15 minutes.

The Therapeutic Sound "Hong"

The practice of the therapeutic Buddhist sound "Hong," the vibrations of which cause the energy of the kidneys to rise up through the body, is indicated to prevent and reverse fatigue, exhaustion, and physical degenerations caused by aging. The sound "Hong" has an invigorating effect on the kidneys, marrow, brain, cerebellum, and genital organs. It is helpful for memory loss and difficulty in concentration.

Sit or stand straight with your hands crossed on the dantian.

Utter the sound "Hong" with great force, making it vibrate in the kidneys, bones, and cranium. The sound should be intense, sustained, and always uttered on the same frequency.

Strengthening the Hearing

Beating the Drums of Heaven ("Golden Marrow")

This exercise is indicated for deafness, auditory disturbances, loss of equilibrium, and eye inflammations.

See Photos 254 to 257. Fold forward the pinna and lobe (the flaps) of both ears and press the palms of your hands against them with your fingers pointing to the back of your head. Press your hands against your ears quite strongly, so that you can no longer hear any outside sound. Cross your index fingers over your middle fingers, then snap your index fingers off your middle fingers to tap your neck. Repeat this snapping procedure 32 times, tapping between the points *Fengfu* (16 DM) and *Yamen* (15 DM, see Figure 8). In cases of audial disturbances such as hissing, ringing, and random sounds in the ears, tap 64 times.

Stimulating the Auditory Canal

This exercise is indicated for tinnitis, migraine headaches, and hearing problems.

Gently introduce your forefingers into the canals of both ears, blocking them well, and place your thumbs on the *Daying* point (5 St) on the lower jaw, your middle fingers on the *Xuanlu* point (5 GB), and your ring fingers on the *Xuanli* point (6 GB, see Figure 10). These last points are located above the temples.

As you inhale, push the auditory canals upward; as you exhale, push them downward. After you have repeated these movements eight times, unplug your ears in a sudden motion while pressing on the tragus, the small cartilaginous protrusion at the front of the ear. You will feel a sensation of great calm.

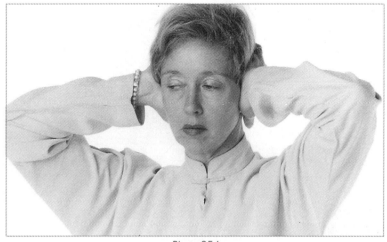

Photo 254

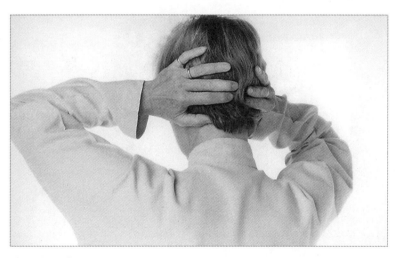

Photo 255

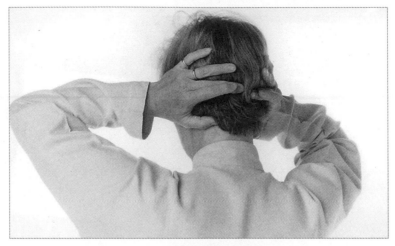

Photo 256

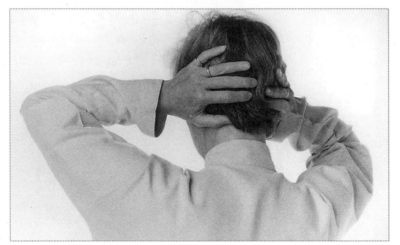

Photo 257

Common Physical Problems of Women

Massaging the Tinggong Point ("Golden Marrow")

This exercise, which is composed of two parts, is indicated for hearing problems, deafness, tinnitis, and toothaches.

Tinggong (19 SI) is the key point of the small intestine meridian (see Figure 10). It is located just in front of the tragus of the ear, in the hollow that forms when you open your mouth very wide.

Part One. Cross your index fingers over your middle fingers and place your middle fingers on both *Tinggong* points, massaging them circularly (see Photo 258). As you inhale, massage upward; as you exhale, massage downward and to the back.

Part Two. As you inhale, cover your ears with the palms of your hands and apply strong pressure for a few seconds; as you exhale, relax the pressure suddenly.

Strengthening the Teeth

Tapping the Teeth 36 Times ("Golden Marrow")

Tap your teeth 36 times in succession, then swallow your saliva 3 times, mentally visualizing its journey to the stomach. The salivary enzymes (called by the Chinese "celestial water") activate digestion and work to prevent tumors of the digestive system.

Rotating the Tongue ("Golden Marrow")

This exercise is indicated for swollen gums, pyorrhea, abnormal development of the tongue, dental problems, dysphonia, and heart problems.

Sweep your tongue over your teeth in a circle, 8 times in one direction and 8 times in the other, up to a maximum of 64 times.

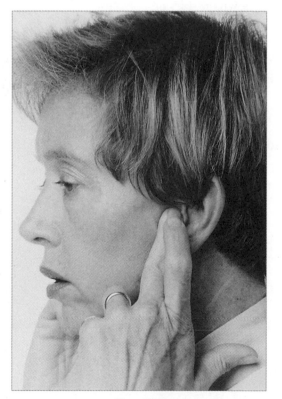

Photo 258

Strengthening the Memory

Combing Your Hair Back ("Golden Marrow")

During this exercise energy flows along the path of the meridians of the bladder, the gall bladder, and the triple heater. The exercise is indicated for high blood pressure and eye problems and improves blood circulation in the brain. It is of particular help to the elderly.

See Photos 259 to 268, which illustrate this exercise. Press the *Jingming* point (1 B, see Figure 4) on the inner corner of the eyelids three or five times. Then making your hands like claws, vigorously comb your hair backward, letting your hands slide down onto your neck until they reach the seventh cervical vertebra just where it juts out, at the *Dazhui* point (14 DM, see Figure 8).

Then slide your hands down along the meridian of the gall bladder, along the sides of the neck and chest and under the armpits, then down the sides of your torso, hips, and thighs. Finally, visualize the qi flowing along the outside of your legs until it reaches the last point of the gall bladder meridian, *Zuqiaoyin* (44 GB, see Figure 18), located at the outer corner of the nail on the fourth toe.

Rotating the Fingers ("Golden Marrow")

For this exercise, see pages 113–116 in this chapter, together with Photos 202 to 213.

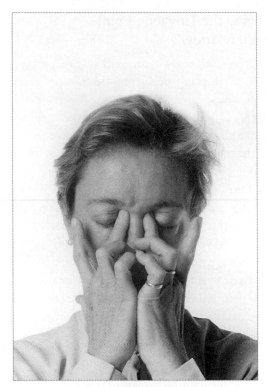

Photo 259

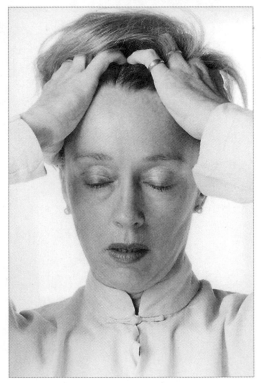

Photo 260

Common Physical Problems of Women

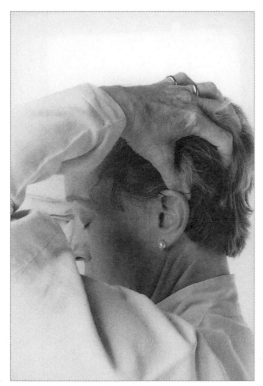

Photo 261

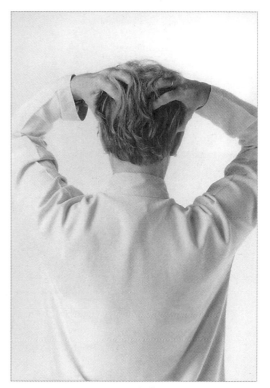

Photo 262

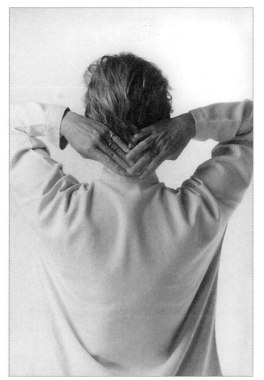

Photo 263

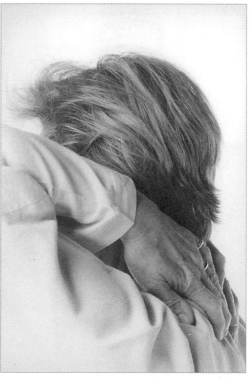

Photo 264

Common Physical Problems of Women

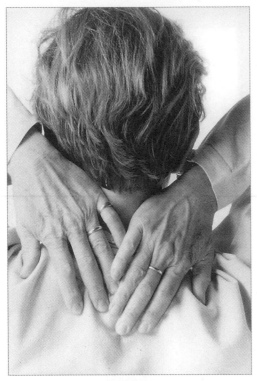

Photo 265

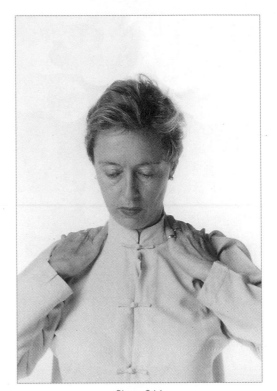

Photo 266

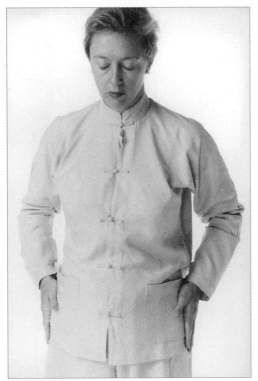

Photo 267

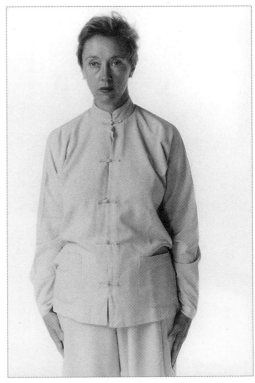

Photo 268

Common Physical Problems of Women

Gynecological Disturbances

How to Regulate Your Cycle and Alleviate Menstrual Pain

Reflexology. To alleviate menstrual pain or in cases of menstrual irregularity, you can first use a foot massage that encourages elimination, working along the path indicated in Figure 20.

You can also circularly massage your ankles around the inner and outer faces of the anklebone, paying particular attention to the half circle just beneath them. Then using both your thumb and index finger, massage the two posterior points of the ankle bone: *Kunlun* (60 B, located between the apex of the outer ankle bone and the Achilles' tendon, see Figure 18) and *Taixi* (3 K, located between the apex of the inner anklebone and the Achilles' tendon, see Figure 18).

Acupressure. Using your fingertips, massage the following pairs of points in a circular motion for two to three minutes: *Hegu* (4 LI, on the back of the hand, see Figure 21), *Sanyinjiao* (6 Sp, see Figure 18), and *Zusanli* (36 St, see Figure 17). Then massage the single point *Guanyuan* (4 RM, located 3 cuns below the navel, see Figure 15) and the pair of *Guilai* points (29 St, located 4 cuns below the navel and 2 cuns from the median line of the womb, see Figure 15).

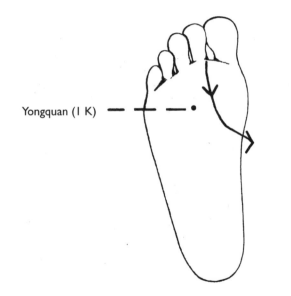

Yongquan (I K)

Figure 20: The point on the foot that alleviates menstrual pain

Moxa for Dysmenorrhea

In cases of overly heavy bleeding, light a stick of moxa and use it to heat the following points for two to three minutes: *Dadun* (1 Lv, see Figure 12), located on the top of the first toe on the outside edge of the distal phalanx, 0.1 cun behind the outside back corner of the toenail, and *Yinbai* (1 Sp, see Figure 12), located 0.1 cun behind the inside back corner of the same nail.

Exercise: Stimulating the Mingmen

This exercise is described in Chapter 1, during the discussion of stimulating the *Mingmen* point.

Pregnancy

To stay in shape during pregnancy—aside from following the diet prescribed by your gynecologist and abstaining from cigarettes and alcohol—it is helpful to follow a gentle program of qigong (incorporating natural, not abdominal breathing) comprising the following exercises:

- Massage of the meridians (see Chapter 4)
- Energetic acupressure of the fingertips (see Chapter 1)
- The nine points of youth (see Chapter 1)

The practice of therapeutic sounds as I have described them can also be very useful, inasmuch as it serves to regulate excesses of emotion. During pregnancy, of course, a woman should try to stay as serene and relaxed as possible, since the child she is carrying in her womb is attuned to—actually participates by osmosis in—her state of mind.

How to Change the Position of the Fetus

To avoid the risk of breech birth, during and after the seventh month of pregnancy you can use burning moxa over the *Zhiyin* point of the foot (67 B, see Figure 18), located at 0.1 cun behind the back outer corner of the nail of the fifth toe. Before doing so, however, you should ask for authorization from your doctor.

The pregnant woman should be lying down while whoever is treating her lights the stick of moxa (see Introduction) and waits for it to burn down a little so that its point assumes a conical shape. It should then be held close to the meridian point, about 1 to 2 centimeters away from the skin (the patient should feel warmth but never burning heat) for about 10 seconds. When the heat becomes too intense, the moxa stick should be raised for a few seconds, then lowered once more. Repeat for 10 to 15 minutes.

Immediately afterward the pregnant woman should remain on the bed, positioned so that she is leaning on her elbows and knees, for about 30 minutes, to allow the fetus to turn comfortably.

Repeat the whole treatment twice if results are not obtained at once.

How to Accelerate Contractions During Birth

Acupuncture is recommended, since it is most effective for this, but you can also use acupressure on the following points:

- *Hegu* (4 LI, see Figure 21)
- *Sanyinjiao* (6 Sp, see Figure 18)
- *Kunlun* (60 B, see Figure 18)
- *Zhiyin* (67 B, see Figure 18)

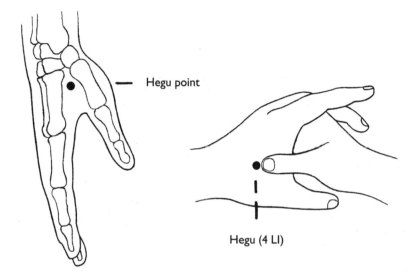

Figure 21: A point on the back of the hand

Hegu point

Hegu (4 LI)

The Fourteen Meridians

Large Intestine Meridian (LI)

Lung Meridian (Lu)

Stomach Meridian (St)

Spleen Meridian (Sp)

Small Intestine Meridian (SI)

Heart Meridian (H)

Bladder Meridian (B)

Kidney Meridian (K)

Triple Heater Meridian (TH)

Pericardium Meridian (P)

Gall Bladder Meridian (GB)

Liver Meridian (Lv)

Du Mai, or Governing Vessel (DM)

Ren Mai, or Conception Vessel (RM)

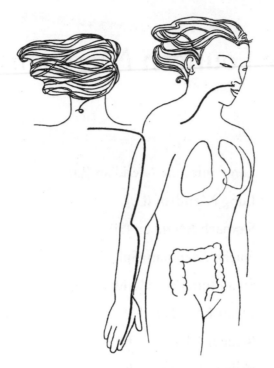

Large Intestine Meridian (LI)

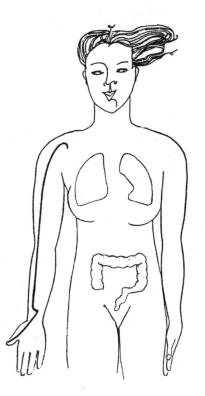

Lung Meridian (Lu)

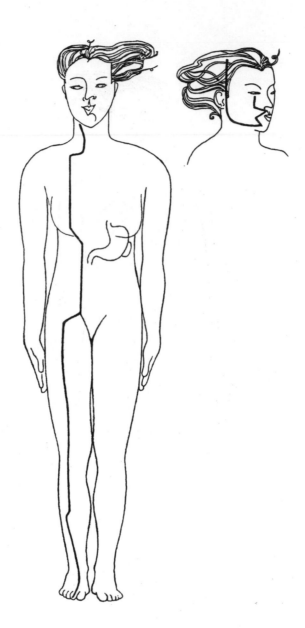

Stomach Meridian (St)

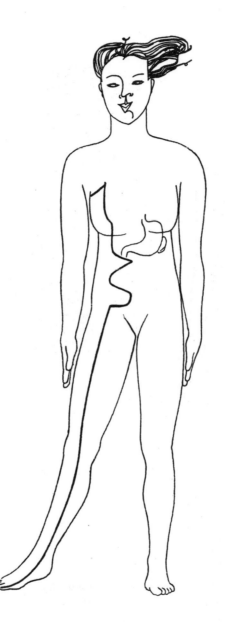

Spleen Meridian (Sp)

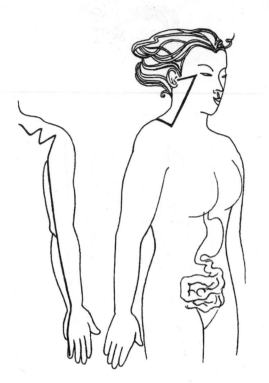

Small Intestine Meridian (SI)

The Fourteen Meridians

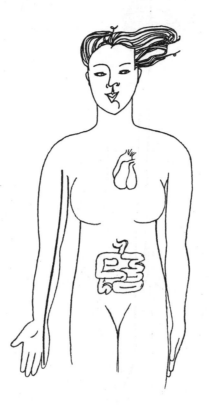

Heart Meridian (H)

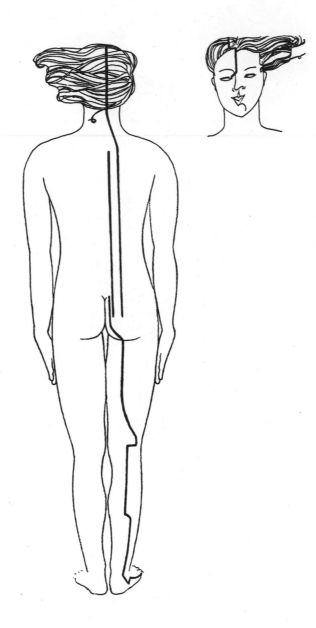

Bladder Meridian (B)

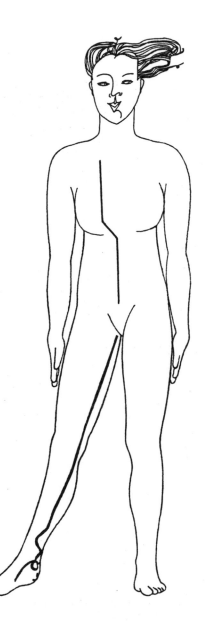

Kidney Meridian (K)

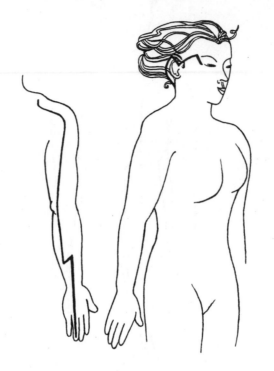

Triple Heater Meridian (TH)

The Fourteen Meridians

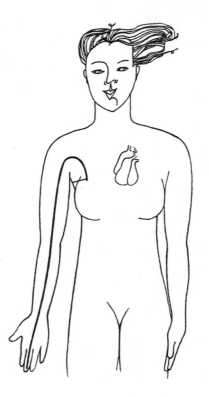

Pericardium Meridian (P)

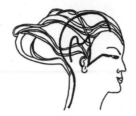

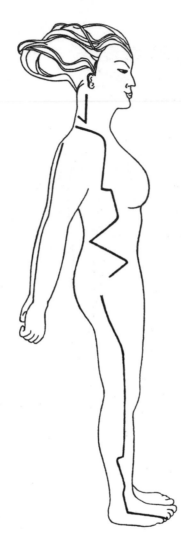

Gall Bladder Meridian (GB)

The Fourteen Meridians

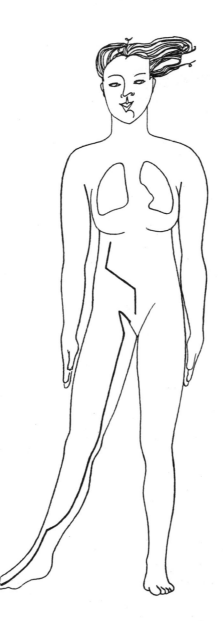

Liver Meridian (Lv)

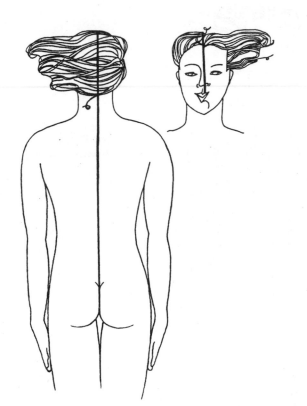

Du Mai, or Governing Vessel (DM)

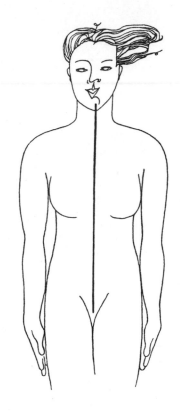

Ren Mai, or Conception Vessel (RM)

The Fourteen Meridians

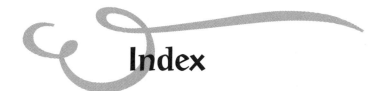

Index